Gastric Sleeve Cookbook

60 Delicious Recipes and Step-By-Step Explanation for Each Stage of Your Recovery from Weight Loss Surgery (Bariatric Surgery Recovery Guide)

Author

Vince Vuong

It is desirable that every patient who has undergone a gastrectomy has undergone a nutritional assessment at a specialized facility. In fact, nutritional support must be personalized in relation to the nutritional status, the clinical history, and the needs of the individual patient as tolerability to foods vary greatly. Therefore, it is emphasized that the information in this book is purely indicative and cannot and should not replace the intervention and the advice of the specialist. Each patient has his own story that deserves to be heard.

TABLE OF CONTENT

INTRODUCTION

The gastric sleeve (or sleeve gastrectomy) outperformed the gastric sidestep as the most performed weight reduction surgery in America in 2013, with 42% of all techniques done broadly being gastric sleeve. This is partly due to the sleeve gastrectomy's amazing weight reduction rates with negligible difficulties.

An appropriate gastric sleeve eating routine will enable you to lose the most weight and maintain it afterwards. Know what you can and can't eat amid each phase of the pre-operation and recuperation process, alongside supper thoughts and patient tips to remain on track.

Patients who pick gastric sleeve surgery lose between 60 percent and 77 percent of their excess body weight within a year of surgery. Similarly, as with all weight reduction, fluctuations come about in light of a few variables which are consistent with post-agent behavioral rules.

In this book, we are going to explain how to face a gastric sleeve diet, which has an important role before and after the surgery, as well as the habits you've got to have.

Chapter 1

What is Gastric Sleeve Surgery?

Gastric sleeve surgery, otherwise called the sleeve gastrectomy, has become a well-known choice for patients looking for superb weight reduction in a direct strategy that doesn't require the upkeep and long-haul intricacy rates of a lap band.

A gastric sleeve is a surgical weight reduction strategy that permanently reduces the size of your stomach by 66%. The technique is performed through a keyhole and is known as a laparoscopic sleeve gastrectomy. A little cut is made in your belly — diminishing scarring and limiting post-surgery recuperation time. The specialist will pass the laparoscope and the instruments required for the surgery through this opening.

After the partial evacuation of your stomach, the rest of your stomach is shut with staples. The procedure is performed under a general soporific and patients can, for the most part, continue ordinary obligations inside half a month. Unlike other weight reduction procedures, like stomach banding, the task is irreversible and does not include implantation of external materials like with a gastric band.

As you will eat less, it is vital that what you do eat gives you the correct supplements that your body requires.

How does this sort of weight loss surgery help?

This method reduces the stomach's capacity and ensures you easily feel full and sated. Additionally, the evacuation of most of the stomach brings about a decrease in the ghrelin hormone, which in turn decreases craving and lets patients feel less ravenous between dinners. This aids weight reduction as the patient eats less and infrequently.

Who can potentially benefit from this method?

In case you are extremely chubby and have a weight file (BMI) of 40, have a BMI of 35 and over, and have depleted every other alternative to get in shape, you might be a decent possibility for a gastric sleeve. Every patient is assessed to decide if they are fit for surgery and whether they fully understand the dangers and duty related to the procedure.

For what reason would it be a good idea for me to consider weight loss surgery?

Excess weight is a major cause for despondency, expanded uneasiness, lessened social acknowledgment, and it negatively impacts on your persona. The aim of a sleeve gastrectomy is to reduce your weight down to a more secure range with the goal that the majority of the related conditions are decreased or dispensed of, prompting a more satisfied presence.

In case you are excessively fat and you can't control your weight through standard means, a laparoscopic sleeve gastrectomy can help you recover.

POTENTIAL BENEFITS TO PATIENTS

Gastric sleeve surgery has the following advantages:

1. May diminish hunger.

2. The craving actuating hormone ghrelin is diminished by evacuating a bit of the stomach, which, to a great extent, is accountable for its generation.

3. Reduced appetite occurs in many patients, though not all.

4. Shorter working time contrasted with gastric sidestep.

5. Does not re-course digestion tracts.

6. No dumping disorders.

7. While a dumping disorder can be an instrument to fortify great dietary patterns, it's exceptionally unsavory.

8. The pylorus stays in place and sugars have sufficient energy to process since the digestive organs stay untouched.

9. No modifications are required. The lap band requires standard alterations (specialist visits).

10. No remote articles are left in the body. The lap band leaves a silicone band around the upper part of your stomach.

11. Weight reduction happens for over a year and a half.

12. Gastric sidestep weight reduction is quick. The larger part of weight reduction happens within the first year.

13. A lap band is slow and requires significant changes to one's way of life for progress. The lion's share of weight reduction happens for more than three years.

Chapter 2

Steps to take before your gastric sleeve surgery

For any planned and elective method, it's fitting to know the angles that you as a patient can or should mull over to make a positive commitment to the advancement of both the intraoperative and postoperative process.

Here, we give you profitable counsel which will assist your involvement with gastric sleeve surgery with being as smooth and positive as can reasonably be expected.

It is a considerable measure of data. However, we think it will be best for you to take these tips as a decent reason for your planning and also having a clearer plan for how to get ready for your gastric sleeve surgery.

Keep close contact with your bariatric specialist

Keeping close contact either specifically with your bariatric specialist or, if nothing else, with the patient facilitator is the premise for the achievement of your gastric sleeve surgery and is crucial for all the accompanying tips that follow.

In the event that what you need is to accomplish the best outcome amid and after your surgery, it's critical that you are as close as possible with the bariatric aggregate since there are numerous imperative perspectives that must be considered as a feature of the arrangement procedure for the task.

This will keep in mind the possible errors that may influence your preparation before and mindset after surgery. Our proposal is that you take on board each suggestion you are given.

Each bariatric deals with their patients distinctively, and it would be difficult to depend on proposals from companions who had the surgery themselves or from discussions with gastric sleeve surgery patients where everybody explains their situation. It merits realizing what others are doing, yet it will be more vital to adhere to the directions of the experts who will be working with you.

Quit smoking before surgery

With their perspective being the end reason to having gastric sleeve surgery is for your health, either on the grounds that you experience the ill effects of stoutness related infections or need to evade them, one point to consider is that if you are a smoker, take this as a defining moment to essentially change those propensities that negatively influence your wellbeing.

Since smoking is detrimental to an individual's wellbeing, and considering that you will undergo a major surgery, the suggestion is that you should also try to stop smoking. This is easier said than done. Yet, we recommend you do your best to quit smoking. Perhaps, you have tried and it can be difficult. However, we recommend you endeavor to abandon it altogether.

The perfect time to stop is a month before surgery, as it will allow your body to "recuperate" from the detrimental effects of smoking, particularly your airways.

During the postoperative period, it is essential not to smoke. This is aimed at minimizing the risks attributed to quick postoperative period recuperation. For example, creating atelectasis (fall of the lung) or pneumonia (lung contamination).

Quitting will also aid the mending process of your entry points and stomach. The least prescribed time to abstain from smoking is a month after surgery.

A complexity that speaks to the most astounding danger and can be expected as a result of not quitting is the probability of a gastric hole. Cigarettes make you susceptible to a diminished blood flow to the majority of your organs, including the stomach, and this causes a drawback in the recuperating process with the likelihood of a fistula (a gap in your stomach) ensuing, which as a rule, requires reoperation.

In this way, in a perfect world you should forsake cigarettes permanently, yet in the event that you don't figure you can change your habits, it is important to abstain from smoking for 30 days prior and 30 days after your surgery.

In case you're a "bad-to-the-bone" smoker, it won't help in the event that you quit smoking the day preceding surgery. Smoking suspension so near the surgery may even be counterproductive in light of the fact that as I talked about already, the body starts to recuperate and the typical elements of the airways begin to recoup and this will make you have more bodily fluid generation.

This does not imply that we recommend that in the event that you don't quit smoking a month prior, it's ideal that you keep on doing so until a couple of hours beforehand.

Of course, it would be counterproductive if, after a successful surgery, you end up creating complexities because of cigarettes.

What to eat before surgery

This subject is dependent on which bariatric assembly you pick. However, the general thought is the same: each patient with a poor weight record ought to experience a preoperative eating regimen, which ought to be given by your bariatric specialist.

For patients who don't require such a preoperative eating routine and can eat regularly before surgery, on the day preceding the method it is prescribed not to eat any large meals after 8 pm and no fluids after 12 pm. Once more, this may fluctuate based upon the specialist you pick.

Additionally, it is essential that after your gastric sleeve surgery, you incorporate a proper eating routine, high in protein, vitamins, and minerals, with the objective of having the ideal healthy condition. Since the surgery itself speaks to a "hostility" to your body, so you should be set up with appropriate nourishing as quickly as possible.

You ought to maintain a strategic distance from:

Soda pops, regardless of the shading since numerous individuals believe that if the drink is clear in shading they are less destructive.

Beverages with caffeine, espresso, sodas, caffeinated drinks, tea, and so on. You can supplant these with decaffeinated and non-carbonated drinks.

Lastly a helpful proposal in connection with sustenance and fluids is that you should begin to "hone" how to ingest fluids with little taste and chew every bite of your nourishment. This will significantly enable you to have better habits after surgery, since the system itself will compel you to do this in the initial couple of weeks, and the need to eat gradually and eat less is vital to losing weight.

The most effective method to get ready mentally before gastric sleeve surgery

The psychological/passionate arrangement is also dependent upon the bariatric gathering. What we propose as a major aspect of the preoperative assessment is that a mental assessment of the patient ought to be performed to establish that there is no contraindication to experience the methodology and to confirm that the patient is rationally fit and prepared to convey every one of the ramifications of such a technique.

Our proposals for this will fluctuate contingent upon the patient. What we look for is to make certain that the patient is completely mindful of the ramifications of having the surgery and has the vital responsibility regarding follow-up therapeutic signs, particularly in the feeling of satisfaction of postoperative eating regimen, all with the objective of limiting the danger of inconveniences and to have normal outcomes in connection to weight reduction.

In a perfect world, the patient ought to know about every one of the advantages and disadvantages of surgery and its dangers. We recommend that their friends and family be associated with the procedure, keeping in mind the end goal is to have them as partners and to get the best help from them including having the ideal conditions at home for the patient's recuperation.

As a recommendation, we encourage you to book a meeting with an advisor who can inform you of the entire procedure. An expert, for example, can help you better understand the progressions that precede and follow your surgery.

Another proposal with respect to a movement you could receive is to compose a journal about your experience. Specialists recommend that our feelings ought to be put on paper. This incorporates your objectives, desires, and your goals for the future after the method. After the surgery, this can enable you to be relaxed in the event that you "release" your feelings in your diary.

Instructions to physically prepare before surgery

A patient's physical readiness before gastric sleeve surgery is generally hard to accomplish as most patients who are looking for bariatric surgery as an answer for their corpulence issue do so on the grounds that their wellbeing status and physical constraints don't enable them to exercise routinely.

Making slight improvements in your daily routine will be helpful prior to the surgery. Exercise consistently before surgery is proposed, with no less than 30 minutes of light exercise every day.

In any case, inability to exercise before surgery would not really create any issues amid the process. The objective is to help your body and mind get used to being dynamic and have the propensity to work out.

Exercise ought not to be strenuous; we simply recommend you to adjust certain basic perspectives: on the off chance that you sit for drawn-out stretches of time, stand up often, walk short distances, abstain from utilizing the lift or escalators, and don't utilize the nearest accessible parking spot to the entryways of the store, but use the most distant accessible spot. If your work and everyday life does not enable you to practice a great deal, take a couple of minutes out of the day to simply walk, have a go at walking your puppy, head off to the recreation center with your children, and so on. All these little changes together add up to a more dynamic life than what you most likely have now and are exceptionally easy to do.

Exercise will help especially by building up a superior lung capacity, which will diminish the odds of respiratory problems in the quick and intervening postoperative period.

A physical change that is really obligatory before surgery is to decrease the size of the liver. This point is clarified in detail in the accompanying posts:

To what extent would it be a good idea for me to eat fewer carbs before my gastric sleeve surgery and what amount of weight would good for me to lose?

Healing Facility Checklist

The rundown of proposed things to bring for your recuperation in the healing facility after surgery can be a lot or little, regarding what you need to take along.

We recommend you take the essentials, particularly in the event that you are coming from a remote place. The general patient experience is that they pack a greater number of things than what they really require for the duration of two evenings in the healing center.

Prescribed rundown by Obesity Free:

Strips to lessen intestinal gas, e.g. Gas-X strips or comparable.

On the off chance that you endure obstructive sleep apnea and have a CPAP machine, it is critical that you carry it with you.

Some sort of oral cream like chapstick and swabsticks like the lemon glycerin swabsticks by Dynarex ®.

Apparel for when you can stroll in the healing center's halls.

Comfortable shoes.

Bring every one of the meds you generally take at home. It is likely you won't require them since they will be dealt with that through the I.V prescriptions given to you amid your stay; however, it is advised to bring them to the clinic

PC, tablet, books, magazines. During your doctor's facility stay, you will presumably feel good enough the day after surgery that you will get exhausted, so we prescribe you to bring things to divert your attention when you're just laying down in your room. What's more, obviously your companion or a relative coming with you will additionally profit on the off chance that you bring things for all the extra time they will have.

Earrings, gems, and so on. This is something you ought to abstain from bringing; notwithstanding on the off chance that you need to wear them, we recommend that you take them off before surgery.

Remote Patients:

In the event that you live in the US, it is likely that you have particular inquiries concerning the things you can or should bring.

Utilize everything examined above. Mexican Pesos: you don't have to change your cash to pesos since in the greater part of the spots you will be during this period accept dollars.

Drinking water: drinking tap water isn't prescribed in Mexico, so we do recommend for you to bring filtered water or whatever other refreshments your partner might want. For your situation, as a patient, don't stress; we will give ice from sterile water, sterile water, and packaged juice. In the event that your partner does not bring along anything to drink, it shouldn't be an issue. Ideally, there will be a lot of safe alternatives to look over in the doctor's facility.

Each remote patient that enters México will be asked to provide their travel permit upon arrival to the USA, so in the event that you don't have it, it is recommended to have this a few weeks or even a very long time before the day of your surgery.

Chapter 3

Gastric Sleeve Diet before the surgery

You should start your gastric sleeve abstain from food around 3 weeks before surgery. At least three weeks prior to surgery, you ought to rehearse a long haul consume less calories. A long haul eating regimen should comprise of for the most part entire, crisp nourishments, and restricted handled sustenance.

CUMIN-SCENTED CABBAGE SALAD

This easy cabbage salad is full of root vegetables and scented with ground cumin.

Preparation Time: 10 minutes

Total time: 10 minutes

Serves 8

INGREDIENTS:

1.   1 head green cabbage, thinly sliced

2.   2 large carrots, sliced into coins

3.   5 scallions (aka green onions), sliced

4.   2 large radishes, sliced

5.   1/4 cup chopped cilantro

6.   1/4 cup apple cider vinegar

7.   1 clove garlic, minced

8.   1/4 teaspoon ground cumin

9.   1/4 teaspoon sweet paprika

10.   1/8 teaspoon fine sea salt

11.   1/8 teaspoon freshly ground black pepper

12.   1/4 cup olive oil

INSTRUCTIONS:

13.   In a large salad bowl combine the cabbage, carrots, scallions, radishes, and cilantro. Toss gently.

14.   In a small jar or bowl, combine the vinegar, garlic, cumin, paprika, salt, and pepper. Add the olive oil and mix well. Toss with salad.

15. Serve immediately. If desired chill and serve within 2 days.

TANGERINE & ROASTED BEET SALAD WITH FETA & PISTACHIOS

This colorful roasted beet salad recipe uses the beet greens too, but you'll likely need more — buy extra beet greens or chard, or even try kale. Serve this healthy dish alongside grilled chicken or pork tenderloin or as an impressive potluck salad.

Preparation Time: 45m
Total time: 1h 45m
serves 4

INGREDIENTS

16. 2 medium beets, trimmed
17. 4 cups chopped beet greens or chard
18. 8 Pixie tangerines or clementines

19. 1 tablespoon sherry vinegar

20. ¼ teaspoon Dijon mustard

21. ½ teaspoon kosher salt, divided

22. Ground pepper to taste 6 teaspoons

23. extra-virgin olive oil, divided

24. ¼ cup crumbled feta cheese

25. ¼ cup coarsely chopped toasted unsalted pistachios

INSTRUCTIONS

Preheat oven to 375°F.

26. Scrub beets well; wrap in foil while still wet and place in a small baking pan. Bake until the tip of a knife slips into a beet easily, 1 to 1¼ hours. Let cool, still wrapped, for 15 minutes. Unwrap and let cool for 10 minutes more. Use a paper towel to rub the skins off. Trim off the ends. Slice the beets into wedges or slices. Rinse and drain beet greens (or chard), leaving a little water still clinging to them; set aside.

27. Grate ½ teaspoon zest from 1 tangerine (or clementine). Slice the ends off all the fruit, then slice off the peel and white pith, following the curve of the fruit. Cut the fruit into segments or slices and set aside. Combine the zest with vinegar, mustard, ¼ teaspoon salt and a generous grinding of pepper in a medium bowl. Whisk in 4 teaspoons oil. Add the sliced beets and toss to coat; let stand for 15 minutes.

28. Heat the remaining 2 teaspoons oil in a large nonstick skillet over medium heat. Add the greens and remaining ¼ teaspoon salt; cook, gently stirring, until just wilted, 2 to 3 minutes.

29. Divide the greens among 4 salad plates. Top with the beets, fruit, feta and pistachios. Drizzle with any remaining dressing.

QUINOA-STUFFED DELICATA SQUASH

With its pretty striped skin and uniform shape, delicata squash is a beautiful vessel for serving up this healthy quinoa stuffing. Serve this recipe as a stunning side dish or a vegetarian main with a big leafy green salad alongside.

Preparation Time: 40m

Total time: 1h 15m

serves 4

INGREDIENTS

Squash

2 small delicata squash (12-14 ounces each), halved lengthwise and seeded

¼ teaspoon salt

¼ teaspoon ground pepper

Stuffing

1 cup water plus 2 tablespoons, divided

½ cup quinoa

⅛ teaspoon salt plus

¼ teaspoon, divided

2 tablespoons butter, divided

1½ cups chopped leek (about 1 large), white and light green parts only

1½ teaspoons chopped fresh thyme or ½ teaspoon dried

⅛ teaspoon freshly grated nutmeg

⅓ cup golden raisins, coarsely chopped

⅓ cup coarsely chopped hazelnuts, toasted

2 tablespoons chopped fresh parsley

INSTRUCTIONS

1. To prepare squash: Preheat oven to 400°F. Coat a baking sheet with cooking spray.

2. Season insides of squash with ¼ teaspoon salt and pepper and arrange cut-side down on the prepared pan. Bake the squash until the flesh is tender but the sides are not collapsing, 20 to 25 minutes total. Reduce oven temperature to 350 degrees.

3.　　To prepare stuffing: Meanwhile, combine 1 cup water, quinoa and ⅛ teaspoon salt in a small saucepan; bring to a boil over medium heat. Cover, reduce heat to a simmer and cook until the quinoa is tender, about 15 minutes. Remove from heat, fluff with a fork and let stand, covered, for 10 minutes.

4.　　Melt 1 tablespoon butter in a medium skillet over medium heat. Add leek and the remaining 2 tablespoons water. Season with thyme, nutmeg and the remaining ¼ teaspoon salt. Cover, reduce heat to low and cook, stirring occasionally, until the leek is tender but not brown, 8 to 10 minutes. Stir in raisins during the last 2 minutes.

5.　　Stir the quinoa, hazelnuts and parsley into the leek mixture. Spoon the quinoa mixture into the squash halves, firmly packing as need. Cut the remaining 1 tablespoon butter into slivers and distribute evenly over the tops. Bake the squash until the stuffing is heated through, about 15 minutes.

6. Make Ahead Tip: Prepare through Step 5 and refrigerate for up to 1 day; reheat in a 350°D oven.

7. Easy cleanup: Recipes that reQuire cooking spray can leave behind a sticky residue that can be hard to clean. To save time and keep your baking sheet looking fresh, line it with a layer of foil before you apply the cooking spray.

ASPARAGUS & BABY KALE CAESAR SALAD

Traditional Caesar salad gets a nutrition and flavor boost with the addition of crisp asparagus and dark, leafy baby kale in this healthy recipe. Use arugula or mixed greens for the salad if baby kale isn't at your market.

Preparation Time: 20m

Total time: 20m

serves 4

INGREDIENTS

¼ cup extra-virgin olive oil

1 large egg yolk

2 tablespoons lemon juice

1 small clove garlic, peeled

¼- ½ teaspoon anchovy paste or ½-1 minced anchovy fillet

¼ teaspoon salt

¼ teaspoon ground pepper

¼ cup grated Parmesan cheese

1 bunch asparagus (about 1 pound), trimmed and very thinly sliced

1 5-ounce package baby kale

Cracked black pepper to taste

INSTRUCTIONS

Combine oil, egg yolk, lemon juice, garlic, anchovy to taste, salt and ground pepper in a food processor (preferably a mini food processor). Process until creamy. Add cheese and pulse to combine.

Toss asparagus and kale in a large bowl. Add the dressing and toss to coat. Season with a generous grinding of pepper.

When a recipe calls for raw eggs, you can minimize the risk of food-borne illness by using pasteurized-in-the-shell eggs. Look for them in the refrigerator case near other whole eggs.

FISH WITH COCONUT-SHALLOT SAUCE

This easy fish recipe with a flavorful garlic, thyme and coconut sauce is perfect for a healthy weeknight dinner. Serve with brown rice, to soak up the creamy sauce, and a green salad with vinaigrette.

Preparation Time: 30m
Total time: 30m
serves 4

INGREDIENTS

3 large cloves garlic, chopped

¾ teaspoon kosher salt, divided

2 tablespoons extra-virgin olive oil, divided

2 tablespoons chopped fresh thyme or 2 teaspoons dried

¼ teaspoon ground pepper, plus more to taste

1¼ pounds mahi-mahi, red snapper or grouper, skinned and
cut into 4 portions

2 tablespoons finely chopped shallot

1 cup 'lite' coconut milk

¼ cup unsweetened coconut chips, toasted

Lime wedges for serving

INSTRUCTIONS

1.   Position rack in upper third of oven; preheat broiler to
       high. Line a baking sheet or broiler pan with foil and
       coat with cooking spray.

2.　Mash garlic and ½ teaspoon salt on a cutting board with a fork to make a thick paste. Combine with 1 tablespoon oil, thyme and ¼ teaspoon pepper. Place the fish on the prepared pan and spread the paste on top of it.

3.　Heat the remaining 1 tablespoon oil in a medium skillet over medium heat. Add shallot and cook, stirring, for 30 seconds. Add coconut milk, increase heat to medium-high and bring to a simmer. Reduce heat to medium-low and simmer until reduced to ¾ cup, about 6 minutes. Season with the remaining ¼ teaspoon salt and pepper to taste.

4.　Meanwhile, broil the fish until just cooked through, 6 to 8 minutes. Spoon the sauce on top, sprinkle with coconut and serve with lime.

5.　For the most up-to-date information about choosing sustainable seafood, go to seafoodwatch.org.

6. Look for thin flakes of dried unsweetened coconut called coconut chips in the produce section or near other coconut in large supermarkets and natural-foods stores. To toast: Place coconut chips or flakes in a small dry skillet over medium-low heat and cook, stirring constantly, until light brown in spots, 4 to 8 minutes.

SALMON & ASPARAGUS FARRO BOWL

In this farro and salmon recipe, salmon is poached in a miso-infused broth with bites of tender asparagus and sautéed leeks. If you use farro that's labeled "pearled," a faster-cooking farro, to make this recipe, start with a full cup of grains and reduce the cooking time to 15 minutes. To clean the leeks, trim off the green tops and white roots and split lengthwise. Place in a large bowl of water and swish around to release any sand or soil. Repeat until no grit remains.

Preparation Time: 40m

Total time: 40m

serves 4

INGREDIENTS

3 cups water

¾ cup farro

1 tablespoon extra-virgin olive oil

2 cups halved and thinly sliced leeks, white and light green parts only

1 bunch asparagus, trimmed and cut into 1-inch pieces

2 cloves garlic, minced

2 cups low-sodium chicken broth or "no-chicken" broth

3 tablespoons white miso

1¼ pounds wild Alaskan salmon fillet, skinned and cut into 1-inch pieces

3 tablespoons very thinly sliced fresh basil ¼ teaspoon pepper

INSTRUCTIONS

1. Combine water and farro in a medium saucepan and bring to a boil over high heat. Reduce heat to medium-low, cover and cook until tender and chewy, about 30 minute Drain.

2. About 15 minutes after you start the farro, heat oil in a large saucepan over medium heat. Add leeks and cook, stirring often, until beginning to soften, about 2 minutes. Add asparagus and garlic; cook, stirring, until the asparagus is bright green, about 2 minutes. Add broth and miso; increase heat to high and bring to a boil. Reduce heat to medium and gently stir in salmon. Simmer for 3 minutes. Remove from heat and stir in basil and pepper.

3. Divide the farro among 4 deep bowls and top with the salmon stew.

4. Look for mild-flavored white (sweet) miso, made with soy and rice, near tofu at well-stocked supermarkets. It will keep in the refrigerator for at least a year.

GRILLED CHICKEN WITH BLUEBERRY-LIME SALSA

One lime does double duty in this healthy chicken recipe. The zest adds a citrus punch to the rub for the chicken, and the lime segments are combined with blueberries for a tart and refreshing salsa. Add more chile if you like it hot.

Preparation Time: 40m
Total time: 2h 50m
serves 4

Ingredients

1 lime
1 tablespoon canola oil
¼ teaspoon salt plus
⅛ teaspoon, divided
¼ teaspoon ground pepper
2 bone-in, skinless chicken breasts, cut in half crosswise

1 cup blueberries, fresh or frozen (thawed), coarsely chopped if large

½ serrano or jalapeño pepper, or to taste, finely chopped

2 tablespoons finely chopped shallot

1 tablespoon chopped fresh cilantro

INSTRUCTIONS

1. Zest lime (reserve the fruit). Combine the zest, oil, ¼ teaspoon salt and pepper in a small bowl. Place chicken in a shallow dish meat-side up and spoon the mixture on top. Cover and refrigerate for at least 2 hours and up to 8 hours.

2. Preheat grill to medium.

3. Oil the grill rack (see Tip). Grill the chicken until an instant-read thermometer inserted in the thickest part without touching bone registers 165°F, 8 to 12 minutes per side. Transfer to a serving plate; let rest for 5 minutes.

4. Meanwhile, slice ends off the reserved lime. With a sharp knife, remove the white pith and discard. Cut the segments from their surrounding membranes and coarsely chop. Combine in a small mixing bowl with blueberries, chile, shallot, cilantro and the remaining ⅛ teaspoon salt, stirring gently. Serve with the chicken.

5. Make Ahead Tip: Marinate chicken (Step 1) for up to 8 hours.

6. Oiling a grill rack before you grill helps prevent foods from sticking. Once the grill is heated, oil a folded paper towel, hold it with tongs and rub it over the rack. (Do not use cooking spray on a hot grill.)

GARLIC-OREGANO GRILLED SHRIMP (CAMARONES ASADA EN ESCABECHE)

Escabeche, a quick pickling of already-cooked food, is a common way of preparing fish and vegetables in Mexico. In this healthy shellfish recipe, the shrimp are grilled first, then infused with flavor from a chile, herb and vinegar marinade. Serve with tortilla shells for tacos, on top of a salad or with toothpicks for an easy appetizer.

Preparation Time: 30m

Total time: 50m

serves 8

INGREDIENTS

¼ cup extra-virgin olive oil plus 1 tablespoon, divided

1 medium white onion, thinly sliced

1 teaspoon dried oregano, preferably Mexican

6 whole black peppercorns

2 dried bay leaves

1 teaspoon kosher salt, divided

2 tablespoons finely chopped fresh serrano or jalapeño peppers (including seeds)

3 medium cloves garlic, thinly sliced

½ cup cider vinegar

32 raw shrimp, peeled and deveined, tails left on if desired

¼ cup coarsely chopped fresh cilantro

INSTRUCTIONS

Heat ¼ cup oil in a large skillet over medium-high heat until it shimmers. Add onion, oregano, peppercorns, bay leaves and ½ teaspoon salt and cook, stirring occasionally, until the onion starts to wilt, 4 to 5 minutes. Add chiles and garlic and cook, stirring frequently, until the garlic is fragrant but not colored, 30 seconds to 1 minute. Remove from heat and stir in vinegar. Transfer to a shallow glass baking dish and let cool while you grill the shrimp.

Preheat grill to medium-high.

Pat shrimp dry. Toss in a bowl with the remaining 1 tablespoon oil and ½ teaspoon salt. Thread the shrimp onto eight 12-inch skewers, leaving a little space between each one.

Grill the shrimp, turning once, until just cooked through, 3 to 4 minutes total.

Remove the shrimp from the skewers and add to the onion marinade, gently stirring to combine. Let marinate, stirring occasionally, for at least 20 minutes or up to 1 hour. Sprinkle with cilantro just before serving.

Make Ahead Tip: Cover and refrigerate the marinade (Step 1) for up to 2 days; marinate grilled shrimp (Step 5) for up to 1 hour.

Equipment: Eight 12-inch skewers

Shrimp is usually sold by the number needed to make one pound. For example, "21-25 count" means there will be 21 to 25 shrimp in a pound. Size names, such as "large" or "extra large," are not standardized, so to get the size you want, order by the count per pound.

Both wild-caught and farm-raised shrimp can damage the surrounding ecosystems when not managed properly. Fortunately, it is possible to buy shrimp that have been raised or caught with sound environmental practices. Look for fresh or frozen shrimp certified by an independent agency, such as the Marine Stewardship Council. If you can't find certified shrimp, choose wild-caught shrimp from North America—it's more likely to be sustainably caught.

MEDITERRANEAN TUNA-SPINACH SALAD

This tuna salad recipe gets an upgrade with olives, feta and a tahini dressing. Served over baby spinach, this is the perfect easy and light lunch or dinner salad.

Preparation Time: 10m
Total time: 10m
serves 1

INGREDIENTS

1½ tablespoons tahini

1½ tablespoons lemon juice

1½ tablespoons water

1 5-ounce can chunk light tuna in water, drained

4 Kalamata olives, pitted and chopped

2 tablespoons feta cheese

2 tablespoons parsley

2 cups baby spinach

1 medium orange, peeled or sliced

INSTRUCTIONS

Whisk tahini, lemon juice and water together in a bowl. Add tuna, olives, feta and parsley; stir to combine. Serve the tuna salad over 2 cups spinach, with the orange on the side.

INDIAN EDAMAME QUINOA BURGERS

This bunless **q**uinoa burger recipe with an easy yogurt sauce is a staff favorite. Experiment with different seasonings in place of the ginger and garam masala, such as garlic and cumin for Middle Eastern flair or garlic and chili powder for a Southwestern spin. Serve with a spinach salad and naan or chapati bread.

Preparation Time: 35m
Total time: 35m
serves 4

INGREDIENTS

½ cup quinoa

1 cup water

8 ounces frozen edamame (about 1½ cups), thawed

3 scallions, chopped, divided

1 large egg

1 tablespoon minced fresh ginger

1¼ teaspoons garam masala

½ teaspoon salt plus

⅛ teaspoon, divided

¼ teaspoon cayenne pepper

2 tablespoons extra-virgin olive oil, divided

¾ cup low-fat plain yogurt

½ cup chopped English cucumber

¼ cup chopped fresh cilantro (optional)

¼ teaspoon ground pepper

1 very large tomato, cut into 4 thick slices

INSTRUCTIONS

1. Combine quinoa and water in a small saucepan. Bring to a boil. Reduce heat, cover and simmer until the water is absorbed, about 15 minutes. Remove from heat and let stand 5 minutes.

2. Transfer the quinoa to a food processor; add edamame, 2 chopped scallions, egg, ginger, garam masala, ½ teaspoon salt and cayenne. Pulse until well

combined. Form into four 3½-inch patties (a generous ½ cup each).

3. Heat 1 tablespoon oil in a large nonstick skillet over medium-high heat; swirl to coat the pan. Reduce heat to medium and add the burgers. Cook until browned on one side, 3 to 4 minutes. Carefully turn them over, swirl in the remaining 1 tablespoon oil and brown the other side, 3 to 4 minutes more.

4. Meanwhile, combine yogurt, cucumber, cilantro (if using), pepper and the remaining scallion and ⅛ teaspoon salt in a bowl. Serve the burgers on a tomato slice with the yogurt sauce.

5. Make Ahead Tip: Individually wrap and freeze cooked burgers for up to 3 months. Unwrap and bake frozen burgers on an oiled baking sheet at 375°F for 20 minutes, turning once.

6. Storage smarts: For long-term freezer storage, wrap your food in a layer of plastic wrap followed by a layer

of foil. The plastic will help prevent freezer burn while the foil will help keep off-odors from seeping into the food.

SEASONED BEEF AND VEGETABLES

Seasoned ground beef and vegetables combine in a symphony of flavors, making a great topping for pasta or rice.

Preparation Time: 10m
Total time: 15m
serves 6

INGREDIENTS

1 tablespoon olive oil
2 cups chopped onions
1 cup chopped celery
1 tablespoon chopped garlic

1 1/3-pound ground beef

2 cups chopped zucchini

1 cup chopped bell pepper

5 ounces sliced mushrooms

2 teaspoons kosher salt

1/2 teaspoon red pepper flakes

freshly ground pepper to taste

INSTRUCTIONS

1. In a large heavy pot, heat the oil until shimmering. Add the onions, celery and garlic. Cook until the onions start to go clear.

2. Add the beef, zucchini, pepper, and mushrooms. Cook, stirring until the vegetables are tender and the meat is no longer pink.

3. Season with the salt, red pepper, and black pepper. Serve immediately.

4.   To freeze: cool mixture completely and place in covered dish. Chill before freezing.

SKILLET-POACHED EGGS WITH SPINACH, PEA TENDRILS, AND LEEKS

Eggs cooked on a bed of spinach with aromatic leeks are a great way to start the day. Serve these skillet eggs for breakfast, lunch, or dinner.

Preparation Time: 5 minutes
Total time: 10 minutes
serves 2

INGREDIENTS:

2 tablespoons salted butter or olive oil
1/2 leek, thinly sliced into half moons
2 cups spinach leaves and pea tendrils combination
salt and freshly ground pepper, to taste

2 eggs

INSTRUCTIONS:

1. Melt the butter or heat the oil in a small skillet. Add the leek and saute until tender, about 3 to 5 minutes.

2. Add the spinach and pea tendrils. Stir gently and cook until slightly wilted. Season to taste with salt and pepper.

3. Move the mixture in the pan to create two small wells. Crack an egg into each well. Add salt and pepper as desired and cover until desired doneness, 3 to 6 minutes.

SPICY ONION JAM

Any type of onion will work for this chile-and-pomegranate-infused jam. Spread crostini with goat cheese and top with the spicy-sweet jam for a quick appetizer or tuck some into a steak taco. If you're a fan of spicy foods, use the full amount of ancho chiles.

Preparation Time: 25m
Total time: 55m
serves 32

INGREDIENTS

2-4 dried ancho chiles, stemmed, seeded and broken into pieces
1 cup pomegranate juice
2 tablespoons extra-virgin olive oil 2 pounds onions, thinly sliced (see Kitchen Tip)
1 tablespoon brown sugar
1 tablespoon distilled white vinegar
½ teaspoon salt

INSTRUCTIONS

1.　Place chiles in a small dry saucepan over medium heat. Cook, stirring occasionally, until fragrant, about 2 minutes. Add pomegranate juice and bring to a boil; cover and remove from the heat. Let stand for 20 minutes. Transfer to a food processor or blender and puree until smooth.

2. Meanwhile, heat oil in a large skillet over medium-high heat. Reduce heat to medium-low, add onions and cook until very soft and lightly browned, about 30 minutes. Add sugar and vinegar and cook until the sugar dissolves, about 1 minute. Increase heat to medium;

3. add the chile puree and cook, stirring occasionally, until thickened, about 4 minutes. Stir in salt.

4. Make Ahead Tip: Cover and refrigerate for up to 1 week.

5. Kitchen Tip: Onions contain a volatile compound called lachrymator that reacts with the fluid in your eyes and makes them water. To chop them without crying, try wearing goggles, burning a candle nearby or

cutting them under cold water. To mellow the bite of a raw onion, soak it for an hour in 1 cup cold water, ¼ cup vinegar and ½ teaspoon salt and then rinse thoroughly.

RASPBERRY-THYME VINEGAR

This beautiful raspberry- and thyme_infused vinegar works well in vinaigrettes. Combine with walnut oil and a pinch of salt and toss with baby spinach and goat cheese for a quick salad. Or stir into a little bit of raspberry preserves and use as a glaze for pork tenderloin. The recipe makes enough vinegar so you'll have extra to decant into a decorative bottle or two to give away as a simple homemade gift.

Preparation Time: 40m

Total time: 40m

serves   1

INGREDIENTS

6 cups white-wine vinegar

3 cups fresh raspberries

12 sprigs fresh thyme

Additional fresh herbs for decoration (optional)

INSTRUCTIONS

1. Wash 3 pint-size (2-cup) heatproof glass canning jars (or similar containers) and their lids with hot soapy water. Rinse well with hot water. Fill a large, deep pot (such as a water bath canner) about half full with water. Place the jars upright into the pot; add enough additional water to cover by 2 inches. Bring the water to a boil; boil jars for 10 minutes. Add the lids to the pot, and then remove the pot from the heat. Let the jars and lids stay in the hot water as you prepare the flavoring and vinegar. (Keeping the jars warm minimizes breakage when filling with hot liquid.)

2. Thoroughly rinse raspberries and thyme with water. Remove the jars from the water bath with a jar lifter or tongs. Divide the raspberries and thyme among the jars. Heat vinegar in a large saucepan to a bare simmer (at least 190°F). Carefully divide the vinegar among the prepared jars, leaving at least ¼-inch of space between the top of the jar and the vinegar. Remove lids from the water bath, dry with a clean towel and screw tightly onto the jars.

3. Store the jars in a cool, dark place, undisturbed, for 3 to 4 weeks. Strain vinegar through cheesecloth into another container until the vinegar looks clear. Repeat as needed until all the sediment from the flavor is removed and the vinegar is clear. Discard all solids and pour the strained vinegar back into to rinsed jars or divide among sterilized decorative bottles. Decorate with a few well-rinsed fresh sprigs of thyme and/or raspberries, if desired. (Decorative raspberries will begin to breakdown after a few weeks in the vinegar and should be removed once they begin to lose their shape and/or color.)

4.   Make Ahead Tip: Refrigerate for up to 1 year.

5.   Equipment: 3 pint-size (2-cup) glass canning jars; cheesecloth

EASY SALMON CAKES

If you are trying to boost your intake of omega-3s, try this simple favorite. It is a great way to use convenient canned (or leftover) salmon. The tangy dill sauce provides a tart balance.

Preparation Time: 30m
Total time: 45m
serves   4

INGREDIENTS

3 teaspoons extra-virgin olive oil, divided
1 small onion, finely chopped 1 stalk celery, finely diced

2 tablespoons chopped fresh parsley

15 ounces canned salmon, drained, or 1½ cups cooked salmon

1 large egg, lightly beaten

1½ teaspoons Dijon mustard

1¾ cups fresh whole-wheat breadcrumbs

½ teaspoon freshly ground pepper

Creamy Dill Sauce, (recipe follows)

1 lemon, cut into wedges

INSTRUCTIONS

1. Preheat oven to 450°F. Coat a baking sheet with cooking spray.

2. Heat 1½ teaspoons oil in a large nonstick skillet over medium-high heat. Add onion and celery; cook, stirring, until softened, about 3 minutes. Stir in parsley; remove from the heat.

3.   Place salmon in a medium bowl. Flake apart with a fork; remove any bones and skin. Add egg and mustard; mix well. Add the onion mixture, breadcrumbs and pepper; mix well. Shape the mixture into 8 patties, about 2½ inches wide.

4.   Heat remaining 1½ teaspoons oil in the pan over medium heat. Add 4 patties and cook until the undersides are golden, 2 to 3 minutes. Using a wide spatula, turn them over onto the prepared baking sheet. Repeat with the remaining patties.

5.   Bake the salmon cakes until golden on top and heated through, 15 to 20 minutes. Meanwhile, prepare Creamy Dill Sauce. Serve salmon cakes with sauce and lemon wedges.

6.   Make Ahead Tip: Prepare through step 3. Cover and refrigerate for up to 8 hours.

7.   To make fresh breadcrumbs: Trim crusts from firm sandwich bread. Tear the bread into pieces and

process in a food processor until coarse crumbs form. One slice makes about ⅓ cup.

8. Easy cleanup: Recipes that require cooking spray can leave behind a sticky residue that can be hard to clean. To save time and keep your baking sheet looking fresh, line it with a layer of foil before you apply the cooking spray.

MUFFIN-TIN CRAB CAKES

We've taken the frying and fuss out of crab cakes by shaping and baking them in muffin tins. For the best taste, look for pasteurized crabmeat in the refrigerator case at your market's fish counter, a better choice than canned varieties. Make It a Meal: Try these cakes with some tangy tartar sauce and coleslaw.

Preparation Time: 20m
Total time: 40m
serves 6

INGREDIENTS

1-pound crabmeat

2 cups fresh whole-wheat breadcrumbs, (see Tip) ½ red bell

pepper, minced

3 scallions, sliced

¼ cup reduced-fat mayonnaise

2 large eggs

1 large egg white

10 dashes hot sauce, such as Tabasco

½ teaspoon celery salt

¼ teaspoon freshly ground pepper

6 lemon wedges, for garnish

INSTRUCTIONS

1.   Preheat oven to 450°F. Generously coat a 12-cup
       nonstick muffin pan with cooking spray.

9. Mix crab, breadcrumbs, bell pepper, scallions, mayonnaise, eggs, egg white, hot sauce, celery salt and pepper in a large bowl until well combined. Divide mixture evenly among muffin cups. Bake until crispy and cooked through, 20 to 25 minutes. Serve with lemon wedges.

10. Make Ahead Tip: Cover and refrigerate for up to 2 days. Reheat in the microwave or serve cold.

11. Tip: To make fresh breadcrumbs: Trim crusts from firm sandwich bread. Tear bread into pieces and process in a food processor until a coarse crumb forms. One slice of bread makes about ⅓ cup crumbs.

SHRIMP CEVICHE

Traditional ceviche consists of raw seafood tossed with an acidic marinade (think: citrus juice or vinegar) that "cooks" the fish. We cook the shrimp before marinating it. This recipe originally appeared on Emeril Green, Emeril Lagasse's cooking show on Planet Green. Lagasse has his own brand of frozen wild American shrimp, which meet strict U.S. environmental standards. The shrimp taste sweet and "they just smell like the sea," according to Emeril. Serve this with tostones (fried plantain chips) or tortilla chips.

Preparation Time: 50m
Total time: 2h 30m
serves   8

INGRIDIENTS

Poaching liquid

2 quarts water
¼ cup kosher salt

Ceviche

1 pound raw shrimp (21-25 per pound), peeled and deveined
Juice of 2 lemons
Juice of 2 limes

Juice of 2 oranges

1 cup diced seeded peeled cucumber (¼-inch dice)

½ cup finely chopped red onion

2 serrano chiles, seeded and finely chopped

1 cup diced seeded tomato

1 avocado, chopped into ½-inch pieces

1 tablespoon roughly chopped cilantro leaves, plus more leaves for garnish

¼ cup extra-virgin olive oil

¼ teaspoon kosher salt

INSTRUCTIONS

1. Combine water and ¼ cup salt in a large saucepan; bring to a boil over high heat. Add shrimp and immediately turn off the heat. Let the shrimp sit until just cooked through, about 3 minutes. Transfer to a cutting board until cool enough to handle, about 10 minutes.

2. Chop the shrimp into ½-inch pieces and place in a medium nonreactive bowl (see Tip). Add lemon, lime and orange juice. Stir in cucumber, onion and chiles. Refrigerate for 1 hour.

3. Stir tomato, avocado, chopped cilantro, oil and ¼ teaspoon salt into the shrimp mixture. Let stand at room temperature for 30 minutes before serving. Garnish with cilantro leaves, if desired.

4. Make Ahead Tip: Prepare through Step 2 and refrigerate for up to 4 hours.

5. Kitchen Tip: A nonreactive bowl or pan—stainless-steel, enamel-coated or glass—is necessary when cooking with acidic foods, such as lemon, to prevent the food from reacting with the pan. Reactive pans, such as aluminum and cast-iron, can impart an off color and/or off flavor.

SAUTEED BRUSSELS SPROUTS WITH BACON & ONIONS

Fresh herbs, onion and bacon pair beautifully with Brussels sprouts. This vegetable loves the cool weather of fall and early winter. If you can find them still attached to the stalk, don't be intimidated—buy them, as they're likely more fresh. All you need to do is slice off each sprout with a paring knife. However, you find them at the market, this is a delicious way to prepare them. Recipe adapted from The Art of Simple Food by Alice Waters.

Preparation Time: 35m
Total time: 35m
serves   10

INGREDIENTS

2½ pounds Brussels sprouts, trimmed
4 slices bacon, cut into 1-inch pieces
1 tablespoon extra-virgin olive oil
1 large onion, diced

4 sprigs thyme or savory, plus

2 teaspoons leaves, divided

1 teaspoon salt Freshly ground pepper to taste

2 teaspoons lemon juice (optional)

INSTRUCTIONS

1. Bring a large pot of water to a boil. If sprouts are very small, cut in half; otherwise cut into quarters. Cook the sprouts until barely tender, 3 to 5 minutes Drain.

2. Meanwhile, cook bacon in a large heavy skillet over medium heat, stirring, until brown but not crisp, 3 to 6 minutes. Remove with a slotted spoon to drain on a paper towel. Pour out all but about 1 tablespoon bacon fat from the pan.

3. Add oil to the pan and heat over medium heat. Add onion and cook, stirring often, until soft but not browned, reducing the heat if necessary, about 4

minutes. Stir in thyme (or savory) sprigs, salt and pepper. Increase heat to medium-high, add the Brussels sprouts, and cook, tossing or stirring occasionally, until tender and warmed through, about 3 minutes. Remove the herb sprigs. Add the bacon, thyme (or savory) leaves and lemon juice, if using, and toss.

4.   Make Ahead Tip: Prepare through Step 1, rinse with cold water; store airtight in the refrigerator for up to 1 day. Finish with Steps 2-3, 15 to 20 minutes before serving.

LEMON & DILL CHICKEN

Fresh lemon and dill create a quick Greek-inspired pan sauce for simple sautéed chicken breasts. Make it a meal: Serve with roasted broccoli and whole-wheat orzo.

Preparation Time: 30m

Total time: 30m

serves   4

INGREDIENTS

4 boneless, skinless chicken breasts, (1-1¼ pounds)

Salt & freshly ground pepper, to taste 3 teaspoons

extra-virgin olive oil, or canola oil, divided

¼ cup finely chopped onion

3 cloves garlic, minced

1 cup reduced-sodium chicken broth

2 teaspoons flour

2 tablespoons chopped fresh dill, divided

1 tablespoon lemon juice

INSTRUCTIONS

1.   Season chicken breasts on both sides with salt and
      pepper. Heat 1½ teaspoons oil in a large heavy skillet
      over medium-high heat. Add the chicken and sear

until well browned on both sides, about 3 minutes per side. Transfer chicken to a plate and tent with foil.

2. Reduce heat to medium. Add the remaining 1½ teaspoons oil to the pan. Add onion and garlic and cook, stirring, for 1 minute. Whisk broth, flour, 1 tablespoon dill and lemon juice in a measuring cup and add to pan. Cook, whisking, until slightly thickened, about 3 minutes.

3. Return the chicken and any accumulated juices to the pan; reduce heat to low and simmer until the chicken is cooked through, about 4 minutes. Transfer the chicken to a warmed platter. Season sauce with salt and pepper and spoon over the chicken. Garnish with the remaining 1 tablespoon chopped fresh dill.

MARMALADE CHICKEN

Orange marmalade and freshly grated orange zest make a deliciously tangy sauce for quick-cooking chicken tenders. Serve with brown rice.

Preparation Time: 20m

Total time: 20m

serves   4

Ingredients

1 cup reduced-sodium chicken broth

2 tablespoons red-wine vinegar

2 tablespoons orange marmalade

1 teaspoon Dijon mustard

1 teaspoon cornstarch

1 pound chicken tenders

½ teaspoon kosher salt

¼ teaspoon freshly ground pepper

6 teaspoons extra-virgin olive oil, divided

2 large shallots, minced

1 teaspoon freshly grated orange zest

INSTRUCTIONS

1. Whisk broth, vinegar, marmalade, mustard and cornstarch in a medium bowl.

2. Sprinkle chicken with salt and pepper. Heat 4 teaspoons oil in a large skillet over medium-high heat. Add the chicken and cook until golden, about 2 minutes per side. Transfer to a plate and cover with foil to keep warm.

3. Add the remaining 2 teaspoons of oil and shallots to the pan and cook, stirring often, until beginning to brown, about 30 seconds. Whisk the broth mixture and add it to the pan. Bring to a simmer, scraping up any browned bits. Reduce heat to maintain a simmer; cook until the sauce is slightly reduced and thickened, 30 seconds to 2 minutes. Add the chicken; return to a simmer. Cook, turning once, until the chicken is

heated through, about 1 minute. Remove from the heat and stir in orange zest.

4.   Tip: Chicken tenders are the virtually fat-free strips of rib meat typically found attached to the underside of chicken breasts. They can also be purchased separately. Four 1-ounce tenders will yield a 3-ounce cooked portion. Tenders are perfect for quick stir-fries, chicken satay or kid-friendly breaded "chicken fingers.

ROAST CHICKEN & FENNEL

With Italian spices, some diced fennel and toasty pine nuts, you'll have a gorgeous supper in no time.

Preparation Time: 30m
Total time: 50m
serves 2

INGREDIENTS

1 large bulb fennel, cored and chopped (3 cups)

5 teaspoons extra-virgin olive oil, divided

2 tablespoons fresh rosemary leaves

1 tablespoon freshly grated lemon zest

2 cloves garlic, quartered

½ teaspoon freshly ground pepper

¼ teaspoon salt

4 chicken drumsticks, (1¼-1½ pounds), skin removed

2 tablespoons pine nuts

2 teaspoons white-wine vinegar

INSTRUCTIONS

1. Preheat oven to 450°F. Toss fennel and 2 teaspoons oil in a 9-by-13-inch baking dish. Bake for 10 minutes.

2. Meanwhile, place rosemary, lemon zest, garlic, pepper and salt together on a cutting board. Rock a chef's knife through the ingredients until they are minced

into a fine paste. Transfer the paste into a small bowl and combine with 1 teaspoon oil. Rub the paste all over drumsticks.

3. Heat the remaining 2 teaspoons oil in a large nonstick skillet over medium-high heat. Add the drumsticks; cook, turning occasionally, until browned on all sides, 4 to 5 minutes.

4. After the fennel has roasted for 10 minutes, stir in pine nuts and place the browned drumsticks on top of the fennel. Return to the oven and bake until the fennel is golden and an instant-read thermometer inserted into the thickest part of a drumstick without touching the bone registers 165°F, 15 to 20 minutes more. Remove the chicken from the pan. Toss the fennel with vinegar in the baking dish, scraping up any browned bits. Serve the fennel with the chicken.

VEGETARIAN TACO SALAD

Nobody will miss the meat in this colorful, zesty vegetarian taco salad. The rice and bean mixture can be made ahead and the salad quickly assembled at mealtime. Recipe by Nancy Baggett for EatingWell.

Preparation Time: 40m

Total time: 40m

serves 6

INGREDIENTS

2 tablespoons extra-virgin olive oil

1 large onion, chopped

1½ cups fresh corn kernels or frozen, thawed

4 large tomatoes

1½ cups cooked long-grain brown rice

15-ounce can black, kidney or pinto beans, rinsed

1 tablespoon chili powder

1½ teaspoons dried oregano, divided

¼ teaspoon salt

½ cup chopped fresh cilantro

⅓ cup prepared salsa

2 cups shredded iceberg or romaine lettuce

1 cup shredded pepper Jack cheese

2½ cups coarsely crumbled tortilla chips

Lime wedges for garnish

INSTRUCTIONS

1. Heat oil in a large nonstick skillet over medium heat. Add onion and corn; cook, stirring, until the onion begins to brown, about 5 minutes. Coarsely chop 1 tomato. Add it to the pan along with rice, beans, chili powder, 1 teaspoon oregano and ¼ teaspoon salt. Cook, stirring frequently, until the tomato cooks down, about 5 minutes. Let cool slightly.

2. Coarsely chop the remaining 3 tomatoes. Combine with cilantro, salsa and the remaining ½ teaspoon oregano in a medium bowl.

3.   Toss lettuce in a large bowl with the bean mixture, half the fresh salsa and ⅔ cup cheese. Serve sprinkled with tortilla chips and the remaining cheese, passing lime wedges and the remaining fresh salsa at the table.

4.   Make Ahead Tip: Prepare through Step 1, cover and refrigerate for up to 3 days; reheat slightly before serving.

5.   To remove corn kernels from the cob, stand an ear of corn on its stem end and slice the kernels off with a sharp knife.

6.   To cook rice, bring 1 cup water and ½ cup long-grain brown rice to a boil in a small saucepan. Reduce heat to low, cover, and simmer at the lowest bubble until the water is absorbed and the rice is tender, about 40 minutes. Remove from the heat and let stand, covered, for 10 minutes. Makes 1½ cups.

MANGO & KIWI WITH FRESH LIME ZEST

Kiwi and mango get a burst of citrus flavor in this easy fruit salad recipe.

Preparation Time: 10m
Total time: 10m
serves   1

INGREDIENTS

1 ripe but firm kiwi, diced
½ cup diced ripe but firm mango
½ teaspoons lime zest

INSTRUCTIONS

Toss kiwi and mango with lime zest. Serve at room temperature or cold.

ROAST PORK, ASPARAGUS & CHERRY TOMATO BOWL

In this healthy grain bowl dinner recipe, hummus may seem like an unconventional dressing ingredient, but here we thin it with some hot water to make a rich, creamy drizzle.

Preparation Time: 35m

Total time: 50m

serves   4

INGREDIENTS

2½ cups water plus 2 tablespoons, divided

1¼ cups bulgur

¾ teaspoon salt, divided

1 pound pork tenderloin, trimmed

1 teaspoon dried marjoram

¼ teaspoon ground pepper

2 tablespoons canola oil, divided

1 bunch asparagus, trimmed and cut into 1-inch pieces

1 large red onion, chopped

1 cup halved cherry tomatoes

½ cup finely chopped fresh parsley

2 teaspoons lemon zest

2 tablespoons lemon juice

¼ cup plain hummus

INSTRUCTIONS

1. Preheat oven to 400°F.

2. Bring 2½ cups water to a boil in a medium saucepan. Remove from heat and stir in bulgur and ¼ teaspoon salt. Cover and let stand until tender, about 20 minutes.

3. Meanwhile, sprinkle pork with marjoram, pepper and ¼ teaspoon salt. Heat 1 tablespoon oil in a large cast-iron or other ovenproof skillet over medium-high heat. Add the pork; cook, turning several times, until browned on all sides, 4 to 6 minutes.

4. Toss asparagus and onion with the remaining 1 tablespoon oil and ¼ teaspoon salt in a medium bowl. When the pork is browned, scatter the asparagus and onion around it. Transfer the pan to the oven and roast until an instant-read thermometer inserted in the center of the pork registers 145°F, 12 to 16 minutes. About 5 minutes before the pork is done, scatter the tomatoes over the vegetables in the pan.

5. Transfer the pork to a clean cutting board and let rest for 5 minutes before slicing. Toss the vegetables with the pan juices.

6. Drain any remaining liquid from the bulgur, then stir in parsley, lemon zest and lemon juice. Combine hummus and 2 tablespoons hot -water in a small bowl. Divide the bulgur among 4 bowls and top with the pork and vegetables; drizzle with the hummus sauce.

APPLE WITH CINNAMON ALMOND BUTTER

With a pinch of cinnamon, this healthy snack goes from basic to brilliant. Be sure to choose an almond butter without any added sugar.

Preparation Time: 5m

Total time: 5m

serves   1

INGREDIENTS

1 medium apple

1 tablespoon smooth almond butter

Pinch of ground cinnamon

INSTRUCTIONS

Core apple and cut into 8 slices. Spread each slice with a little almond butter and sprinkle with cinnamon.

CREAMY GARLIC PASTA WITH SHRIMP & VEGETABLES

Toss a garlicky, Middle Eastern-inspired yogurt sauce with pasta, shrimp, asparagus, peas and red bell pepper for a fresh, satisfying summer meal. Serve with: Slices of cucumber and tomato tossed with lemon juice and olive oil.

Preparation Time: m
Total time: 20m
serves   4

INGREDIENTS

6 ounces whole-wheat spaghetti 12 ounces peeled and deveined raw shrimp, cut into 1-inch pieces
1 bunch asparagus, trimmed and thinly sliced
1 large red bell pepper, thinly sliced

1 cup fresh or frozen peas

3 cloves garlic, chopped

1¼ teaspoons kosher salt

1½ cups nonfat or low-fat plain yogurt

¼ cup chopped flat-leaf parsley

3 tablespoons lemon juice

1 tablespoon extra-virgin olive oil

INSTRUCTIONS

1. Bring a large pot of water to a boil. Add spaghetti and cook 2 minutes less than package directions. Add shrimp, asparagus, bell pepper and peas and cook until the pasta is tender and the shrimp are cooked, 2 to 4 minutes more. Drain well.

2. Mash garlic and salt in a large bowl until a paste forms. Whisk in yogurt, parsley, lemon juice, oil and pepper. Add the pasta mixture and toss to coat. Serve sprinkled with pine nuts (if using).

3.   Both wild-caught and farm-raised shrimp can damage the surrounding ecosystems when not managed properly. Look for shrimp certified by an independent agency, such as Wild American Shrimp or Marine Stewardship Council. If you can't find certified shrimp, choose wild-caught shrimp from North America—it's more likely to be sustainably caught.

4.   To toast pine nuts, place in a small dry skillet and cook over medium-low heat, stirring, until fragrant, 2 to 4 minutes.

BEET & SHRIMP WINTER SALAD

This healthy dinner salad recipe gets its staying power from protein-packed shrimp and fiber-rich barley. With a simple red-wine vinaigrette, this quick salad makes just one serving but is easy to double or triple. Look for precooked beets with other prepared vegetables in the produce department.

Preparation Time: 15m

Total time: 15m

serves   1

INGRIDIENTS

Salad

cups lightly packed arugula

1 cup lightly packed watercress

1 cup cooked beet wedges

½ cup zucchini ribbons

½ cup thinly sliced fennel

½ cup cooked barley

4 ounces cooked, peeled shrimp, tails left on if desired

Fennel fronds for garnish

Vinaigrette

2 tablespoons extra-virgin olive oil

1 tablespoon red- or white-wine vinegar

½ teaspoon Dijon mustard

½ teaspoon minced shallot

¼ teaspoon ground pepper

⅛ teaspoon salt

INSTRUCTIONS

1. Arrange arugula, watercress, beets, zucchini, fennel, barley and shrimp on a large dinner plate. Whisk oil, vinegar, mustard, shallot, pepper and salt in a small bowl, then drizzle over the salad. Garnish with fennel fronds, if desired.

2. To make zucchini ribbons, thinly shave whole zucchini lengthwise with a vegetable peeler.

3. Go for sustainably raised shrimp. Look for fresh or frozen shrimp certified by an independent agency, such as the Marine Stewardship Council. If you can't find certified shrimp, choose wild-caught shrimp from

North America; it's more likely to be sustainably caught.

4.   Give grains a cooldown: To cool grains down quickly, spread them out on a foil-lined baking sheet. The surface area helps speed cooling, while the foil prevents any residual flavors on the pan from seeping in.

CRAB ROLL

This healthier take on a lobster roll uses crab because it's usually easier (and less expensive) to buy. But by all means use lobster if you prefer. Serve with coleslaw and an ice-cold beer.

Preparation Time: 20m

Total time: 20m

serves   4

INGREDIENTS

¼ cup low-fat mayonnaise

1 tablespoon freshly grated lemon zest

3 tablespoons lemon juice

10 dashes hot sauce, such as Tabasco

½ teaspoon freshly ground pepper

⅛ teaspoon salt

¼ cup finely chopped shallot

¼ cup finely chopped celery

¼ cup thinly sliced fresh chives, divided

12 ounces cooked crabmeat (about 2 cups; see Tip), drained
if necessary, any shells or cartilage removed

8 leaves red or green leaf lettuce

4 whole-wheat hot dog buns (toasted, if desired)

INSTRUCTIONS

1.   Whisk mayonnaise, lemon zest, lemon juice, hot sauce,
      pepper and salt in a medium bowl. Thoroughly mix in

shallot, celery and 3 tablespoons chives. Mix in crab very gently so it doesn't break up too much.

2. Line each bun with lettuce and divide the crab filling among the buns. Garnish with the remaining 1 tablespoon chives.

3. Make Ahead Tip: Cover and refrigerate the crab filling (Step 1) for up to 1 day.

4. Tip: Crabmeat (already removed from the shell) can be purchased canned, in shelf-stable pouches, frozen or pasteurized. Pasteurized usually has the best flavor; look for it in the fresh seafood section of the market. Crab from the U.S. and Canada are both considered good choices for the environment. If you live in an area known for crab, you may be able to get freshly cooked crabs at the seafood counter of your local market.

8 LAYER TACO SALAD

This gorgeous and colorful 8-layer taco salad recipe is made healthier by using ground turkey in place of beef, adding Greek yogurt and bumping up the amount of vegetables. Serve this salad in a clear glass bowl and you'll have an eye-catching party-worthy dinner or potluck side in just 30 minutes.

Preparation Time: 30m
Total time: 30m
Serves 6

INGREDIENTS

1 tablespoon canola oil

1 pound 93%-lean ground turkey

2 tablespoons chili powder

½ teaspoon salt, divided

1 avocado, pitted

½ cup nonfat plain Greek yogurt

1½ cups crumbled unsalted tortilla chips

1 cup prepared salsa

1 15-ounce can pinto beans, rinsed

5 cups thinly sliced romaine lettuce

½ cup shredded Mexican cheese blend

1 medium tomato, chopped

INSTRUCTIONS

1. Heat oil in a large skillet over medium-high heat. Add turkey, chili powder and ¼ teaspoon salt. Cook, stirring and breaking up lumps, until cooked through, about 5 minutes.

2. Meanwhile, mash avocado, yogurt and the remaining ¼ teaspoon salt in a small bowl with a fork until smooth.

3. Transfer the turkey and any juice from the pan to a serving bowl. Layer chips, salsa, beans and lettuce over

the turkey. Spread the avocado mixture over the lettuce. Top with cheese, then tomato.

TOMATO SOUP

This simple tomato soup is perfect paired with your favorite grilled cheese sandwich. Make a double batch and freeze the extra for rainy-day emergencies.

Preparation Time: 25m

Total time: 35m

serves   8

INGREDIENTS

1 tablespoon butter

1 tablespoon extra-virgin olive oil

1 medium onion, chopped

1 stalk celery, chopped

2 cloves garlic, chopped

1 teaspoon chopped fresh thyme or parsley

1 28-ounce can whole peeled tomatoes, with juice

1 14-ounce can whole peeled tomatoes, with juice

4 cups reduced-sodium chicken broth, "no-chicken" broth or
vegetable broth

½ cup half-and-half (optional)

½ teaspoon salt freshly ground pepper to taste

Chapter 4

Feeding after a gastric sleeve surgery

Getting fitter truly can be a decisive circumstance, especially for those individuals who are very unfit. Time is of the essence and the longer it takes to lose the weight, the more noteworthy the hazard to their wellbeing. Thus, gastric sleeve surgery might be the best choice. On the off chance that you are thinking about this method, you might want to find out about the recuperation procedure; this article on gastric sleeve post operation can help.

This methodology has been accessible for a considerable length of time; though there are a few dangers, as with all surgeries, they are negligible and uncommon. The most well-known issue is the living changes they should make. These progressions can be testing, which is the reason most patients are given a considerable amount of pre-operation guidance, with the goal that they completely comprehend what they should confer themselves to.

The vast majority comprehend the essential idea of gastric sleeve: your stomach is made smaller so you can eat little amounts for sustenance at one sitting. Thus, clearly, a standout amongst the most intense changes will be a drastically diminished sustenance consumption at every feast.

Other post-operation life changes may not appear to be so evident; for example, how you can never again eat a great deal of high-sugar and high-fat substances. Eating excessively this kind of food can prompt blacking out since it will be retained considerably more rapidly than it would have been before the surgery when your stomach actually had more space.

When you are eating less, you are also drinking less, which implies that you should savor water, little sums, during your time to stay away from thirst.

While everybody is unique and every individual outcome will fluctuate, by and large, many patients will lose up to 50% of their additional weight inside the initial half year after surgery. From between six months to two years, the measure of weight reduction will be as high as 70%. Following two years post operation, the normal weight reduction tends to level off at around 80%. It's extremely extraordinary for somebody to lose 100% of their excess fat, so a few people will assert that this kind of surgery isn't effective.

Only the individual can judge the accomplishment for themselves, however, my thought would be that on the off chance that somebody is excessively fat and says something overabundance of 300 lbs, they would be excited to lose 60 - 80% of their extra weight!

In the event that you are extremely overweight and you are desperate to get yourself to a more reasonable weight, you might need to investigate gastric sleeve surgery. This is a suitable path for you to take control of your weight more rapidly than simply a good eating regimen and exercise. Your gastric sleeve post-operation way of life will be unique, but if you're not willing to roll out huge improvements to your way of life the procedure won't work for you. This article has given you a short outline and now you have an idea of what's included, your specialist will answer whatever remains of your inquiries.

Total or subtotal gastrectomy may cause a significant loss of body weight, mainly due to a reduction in diet, often caused by the rapid feeling of satiety perceived after taking a few bites of food. This symptom is a frequent complaint by patients, especially in the first months after surgery. Recent studies have made it possible to clarify that at the basis of the eating disorder, there could also be an altered production of hormones by the gastrointestinal tract. The nutritional intervention in the gastrectomised patient, therefore, aims to:

1. prevent weight loss and malnutrition by default;
2. promote tissue healing after surgery;
3. supplement the nutritional deficiencies caused by the removal of the stomach;
4. place the residual portion of the gastrointestinal apparatus under conditions of physiologically replacing functions not pertinent to it;
5. strengthen the immune system;

6.   eliminate, or at least reduce the symptomatology
      caused by the different post-gastrectomy syndromes.

Below are some general indications that can help
gastrectomized patients to feed themselves properly and
adequately to their condition:

1.   Consume at least 6 meals a day, consisting of small
      amounts of food, trying to favor foods with higher
      nutritional value.
2.   Chew each bite long and slowly, so that the digestion
      process starts at the level of the mouth.
3.   During the meal, maintain an upright position because
      this facilitates the progression of food. Do not lie
      down immediately after meals to avoid reflux.
4.   Limit the intake of liquids during meals, taking care to
      drink 1-1.5 liters of liquids (water, tea, chamomile,
      herbal tea, etc.) during the day.
5.   Consume foods rich in calcium and vitamin D (fish at
      least once a week and milk or dairy products at least
      once a day).

6. Keep a record of the foods that cause disturbances through a food diary, and then possibly exclude them from the diet.

7. In the presence of biliary reflux, it is important that you do not spend much time between a snack and the other (maximum 1 hour and a half). In fact, food in the intestine neutralizes bile and prevents regurgitation. Since bile regurgitation often occurs at night, it is advisable to sleep with 2-3 cushions under the shoulders in order to avoid the horizontal position; it could also be useful to eat a small snack before going to sleep.

The gastrectomy can cause malabsorption; that is, it can reduce the capacity of the intestine to absorb nutrients: about 10% of patients have cramping pains and steatorrhea. For this reason, it is often necessary to check and integrate any fat-soluble vitamins deficiencies. In the presence of diarrhea and steatorrhea, it may be useful to reduce the consumption of fat. It's recommended to divide the diet into small and frequent meals (6-7 per day) and to strictly adhere to this scheme. If the steatorrhea persists, it is useful to introduce

MCT oil into the diet. MCT oil, available in pharmacies, is more easily absorbed than common food oils such as olive oil. However, it is devoid of flavor, does not bring all the fatty acids that are essential for the body, and must be consumed raw. When possible, it is useful to prepare a mixture consisting of 70% MCT oil and 30% of a tasty olive oil to be used raw, in order to give food a more pleasant taste.

If oral feeding proves to be insufficient for caloric-nutritional needs and cannot be corrected by natural nutrition, it should be supplemented with suitable products or replaced with artificial nutrition. Oral nutritional supplements may be used, which, due to their different characteristics of composition, consistency and taste can meet most of the nutritional needs, according to the doctor's instructions and the patient's preferences. Oral nutritional supplements should be taken under the supervision of the nutritionist doctor.

Depletion syndrome

The depletion syndrome, which doctors often refer to using the English term 'dumping syndrome', occurs when the food bolus is rapidly introduced into the small intestine, triggering gastrointestinal and/or vasomotor symptoms. 25-50% of patients undergoing gastric surgery suffer from it, 5-10% of whom develop clinically relevant symptoms.

Symptoms occur during the first three months of surgery and may persist for one year. There are two forms of dumping syndrome, one early and one late. The early form manifests itself 10-30 minutes after meals and includes gastrointestinal and vasomotor symptoms (abdominal pain, nausea, vomiting, diarrhea, headache, vasodilation and redness of the skin, asthenia, and lowering of blood pressure). It derives mainly from the fast flow of food into the small intestine, which determines its rapid and sudden relaxation. The late form occurs 1-3 hours after a meal with predominantly vasomotor symptoms (sweating, weakness, confusion). It is linked to the alteration of blood sugar levels. Due to the lack of the stomach, the sugar is absorbed too quickly in the small intestine. This symptomatology can usually be aggravated by the intake of sweet foods or sugary drinks.

However, these episodes should not create excessive alarm: abdominal pain does not indicate any damage and normally disappears in about 30-60 minutes. If the symptom is early, careful diet assessment is needed, which will limit simple sugars by increasing complex sugars and separating solid foods from liquids. Even the presence of small meals, which include both protein and fat, can help reduce the incidence of early dumping syndrome. If the symptom is late, it usually resolves with the ingestion of complex sugars or minimal amounts of simple sugars and refined carbohydrates at each meal, always consuming liquid and solid foods separately. It is also good to avoid eating foods that are too hot or too cold.

Food to be preferred

1. Complex carbohydrates: pasta, rice, bread. Prefer dry first courses, seasoned with simple sauces (tomato, vegetable sauces).
2. Meat: discard visible fat and poultry skin.
3. Fresh or frozen fish.
4. Cold cuts such as cooked/raw ham (always defatted), bresaola.
5. Vegetables, fresh or frozen, varying the quality.

6. Milk: preferably whole, starting to take it in small quantities. If not tolerated, try milk with high digestibility.

7. Yogurt: take at least one portion (one jar) a day, preferring those made from natural whole milk.

8. Extra virgin olive oil.

9. Butter.

Food not recommended

1. Simple sugars: sugar, jam, honey, etc.

2. Sweets in general and in particular those prepared with creams, chocolate, ice cream.

3. Ready sauces such as mayonnaise, mustard etc.

4. Coffee, strong tea, fizzy drinks (like orange juice, Coca-Cola etc.).

5. Wholemeal or soy flours and foods prepared with these ingredients (wholemeal bread and pasta, wholemeal crackers, soya bread, etc.).

6. Fatty parts of meat and boiled meat as it is difficult to digest.

7.   Fatty fish (eel, mullet, moray eel, lobster) and fish preserved in oil.

Chapter 5

Phases of the gastric sleeve diet

There are five standard phases of the postoperative eating routine for gastric sleeve:

Clear Liquids Diet –Stage 1 (while in healing center).

Protein-Based Liquids –Stage 2 (2-3 days post surgery, 2-week length).

Pureed Foods –Stage 3 (day 15, weeks 3 and 4).

Delicate Foods –Stage 4 (a month 5 and 6).

Normal Foods –Stage 5 (week 7 and past).

Each individual ought to talk about points of interest of an energizing pre-activity like eating less with their specialist, since the correct eating routine differs from individual to individual.

Clear Liquids Diet –Stage 1 (while in healing center)

Stage 1 of the gastric sleeve eating routine more often than not goes on for about seven days after surgery. Amid this time, individuals ought to consume just clear fluids.

Staying hydrated after surgery can speed the recuperation process and help with difficulties, for example, queasiness and heaving.

While it can be difficult to adhere to a reasonable fluid eating regimen, the vast majority feel next to zero yearning in the days instantly following their surgery. They ought to likewise abstain from devouring:

- Juiced drinks, for example, tea and espresso.
- Sugary beverages, for example, natural fruit juice.
- Carbonated beverages.
- Pop.

Rather, individuals should drink sans sugar clear fluids. Notwithstanding no less than 8 glasses of water for every day, a reasonable fluid eating regimen can include:

- Jello.
- Juices.
- Decaf tea or espresso.
- Sans sugar popsicles.

Protein-Based Liquids –Stage 2 (2-3 days post surgery, 2-week length)

In stage 2, a sans sugar protein powder ought to be added to the eating routine.

Seven days to 10 days following surgery, the vast majority who have had gastric sleeve surgery start to get eager once more.

During this stage, they change to a fuller fluid eating regimen that is rich in protein. The objective ought to be to eat an assortment of restorative supplements, yet to maintain a strategic distance from sugary nourishments and substances with low nutritious value.

Nourishments to maintain a strategic distance from ought to include:

- Sugary nourishments.
- High-fat nourishments, for example, full fat yogurt.
- Stout nourishments, for example, vegetable soup.

Someone in stage 2 should keep drinking loads of water and fuse protein into their eating routine by drinking protein powder. The protein powder ought to be sans sugar and blended with clear or full fluid.

The point ought to be to expend 20 grams (g) of protein every day. Admission ought to be restricted to ½ measure of fluid per supper. Without sugar substances, you can incorporate the accompanying:

- Thin soups, including creamed soups.
- Sans sugar pudding, frozen yogurt, or sorbet.
- Weakened juice.

118

- Moment breakfasts with no additional sugar.
- Soft noodles in soup.
- Without sugar non-fat dessert or yogurt.
- Low-sugar fruit purée weakened with water.

Towards the end of the second week or toward the start of the third week, it is okay for somebody to start including thicker, pureed substances. They should keep maintaining a strategic distance from sugar and high-fat substances.

Notwithstanding the nourishments that were safe to eat before, it is currently safe to consume:

- Greek yogurt.
- Diminished oats.
- Squashed sweet potatoes.
- Pureed potatoes.
- Canned, pureed chicken or fish.
- Child nourishments.
- Smoothies and pureed nourishments, as long as there is low or no sugar.

- Fried eggs.
- Pureed whitefish.

Through this stage, individuals should go for 60g to 80g of protein for each day. Greek yogurt, eggs, and fish are rich in protein. To feel full and to guarantee satisfactory protein admission, protein can be eaten as the initial segment of the supper.

Every supper ought to incorporate close to ½ measure of fluids, which means it will be important to eat numerous small dinners.

Pureed Foods –Stage 3 (day 15, weeks 3 and 4)

The change to stage 3 may necessitate including supplement thick delicate nourishments, for example, fried eggs.

Individuals who have had gastric sleeve surgery change to delicate nourishments amid stage 3 of their eating routine regimen should keep eating 60g to 80g of protein every day and stay all around hydrated. It is recommended to eat everything on the pureed substances eating regimen, however, abstain from eating the following:

- Sugary nourishments.
- Bread.
- Skin and seeds from vegetables and natural products.
- Greasy nourishments, particularly oils and spread.
- Extreme, crude vegetables.
- White pasta and rice.

High-protein. Supplement thick delicate foods to bolster fullness and speed up recuperation. A few choices include:

- Low-fat shop meat.
- Delicate fish.
- Low-fat cheddar.
- Eggs, including mixed, poached, or hard-boiled.
- Relaxed vegetables.
- Soups, incorporating those with a few lumps.

It is important to keep drinking a daily protein shake and to confine caffeine to only 1 espresso for each day if permitted by a specialist.

Delicate Foods –Stage 4 (a month 5 and 6)

Around a month after surgery, it is okay for somebody to progress to heavy food. Individuals keen on attempting a gastric sleeve eating regimen can receive organize 4 to endeavor to get more fit.

Everybody should keep drinking a protein shake, and get 60g to 80g of protein for each day. They should stay hydrated, however, quit drinking 30 minutes before their supper.

Taking a daily bariatric multivitamin, as prescribed by a specialist, can likewise be a good piece of this stage. The regimen should focus on adhering to three little suppers for each day and two little bites. Once more, eating sugary or heavily processed low-fiber food ought to be dodged.

Substances to eat

It is now all right to eat most kinds of substances. They should keep eating protein-rich substances from stage 3, and also various foods, for example:

- Low-fat curds.
- Angle.
- Lean meats.
- Vegetables.
- Little amounts of organic product.

Substances to maintain a distance from

Abstain from getting calories from drinks. This influences individuals to feel less fulfilled than solid food does and can cause nutritional shortfalls. Some other different foods to dodge ought to include:

- Bread and white grains.
- Sugary bites.
- Bundled substances, for example, potato chips.
- Cooking oils.

- Fricasseed nourishments.

- Soft drinks.

- Treats.

- High-calorie substances.

Regular Diet After Surgery –Stage 5 (week 7 and past)

A run-of-the-mill supper for a bariatric surgery eating regimen incorporates protein-rich substances, for example, lean meat, eggs, beans, low-fat dairy items, and high-fiber foods including vegetables and organic products.

Chapter 6

30 Healthy recipes to maintain your weight after surgery

THAI CHICKEN WITH SPICY "PEANUT" SAUCE

A Thai-inspired stir-fry sounds innocent enough (veggies! meat! dairy-free!), but it can be a minefield of Whole Diet no-no's, such as soy sauce, honey, and peanut butter. This recipe gets around those roadblocks, subbing in coconut amino's for the soy, a mashed date for sweetness, and sunflower butter as a vitamin E-rich replacement for the peanutty stuff.

INGREDIENTS

1 date

Water

1 garlic clove, pressed

1 T fresh ginger, finely grated

¼ C sunflower butter

Juice of ½ lime

4 T coconut amino

1 T sesame oil

⅛ tsp salt

Red pepper flakes

4 T olive oil

1 lb. chicken tenders

Salt

Pepper

2 medium zucchinis, spiralized

1 handful of carrot shreds

2 sweet peppers, thinly sliced

Sesame seeds

Cilantro, chopped

INSTRUCTIONS

1.   Put the date in a small cup and add enough water to complete cover date. Microwave on high for 1 minute and allow to soak until the date is needed later.

2.   In a small bowl, whisk together garlic, ginger, sunflower butter, lime juice, coconut amino, sesame oil, and salt.

3.   Remove date from the water. Cut pits out of date and discard. With a fork, smash date until it turns into a paste. Whisk date pastes with the rest of the "peanut" sauce.

4.   Add a dash of red pepper flakes to the sauce, enough to add as much heat as preferred.

5.   In a skillet warm 2 T of olive oil over medium-high heat. Add chicken tenders and sauté on each side for 3-4 minutes or until cooked thoroughly. Remove chicken from skillet and set aside to rest and cool.

6.   In the same skillet, add the remaining 2 T of olive oil. Toss zucchini, carrot shreds and sweet peppers in the oil. Stir constantly with tongs and allow to cook for 2 minutes, just long enough to warm the vegetables thoroughly and slightly soften.

7.   Dice chicken and toss with the veggie noodles. Stir in the sauce just before serving.

8.   Garnish with sesame seeds and cilantro.

ROASTED LEMON CHICKEN WITH POTATOES AND ROSEMARY

Already a pretty clean meal, the classic chicken and potato dish didn't need too much tweaking to become Whole compliant. Translation: It's a great way to ease yourself into the plan. Spruce up the protein with a spritz of lemon and the carbs with garlic and rosemary. You've got a succulent dinner that'll make you forget you gave up anything at all.

INGREDIENTS

8-10 pieces of your favorite cut of chicken - skin on bone in

1 lbs. baby red potatoes

1/2 in onion - cut large pieces

2 lemons 1 sliced and 1 juiced

1/3 cup olive oil

2 cloves garlic, minced

1 Tablespoon fresh Rosemary plus sprigs for garnish

1/2 teaspoon crushed red pepper flakes

1 1/2 teaspoon salt

1/2 teaspoon fresh ground pepper

INSTRUCTIONS

1.   Preheat oven to 400 degrees F.

2.   Spray a glass 13-in. x9-in. baking dish with cooking spray. Arrange chicken pieces (skin side up), potatoes, sliced onion and lemon slices evenly in pan.

3.   In a small bowl, whisk together lemon juice, olive oil, garlic, rosemary, crushed red pepper flakes, salt, and pepper.

4.   Pour mixture over chicken, making sure all the chicken is covered. Toss a bit if necessary.

5. Sprinkle generously with additional salt and pepper.

6. Bake uncovered for about 1 hour, or until chicken and potatoes are fully cooked.

CHICKEN BALANCE BOWL

This fresh bowl has all our salad favorites; chicken, sweet potato, and avocado; and a sauce so good you'll want to make extra and keep it in the fridge. (Just double-check that the tahini you go with has no added sugar so it's Whole Diet approved.) A delicious dinner whipped up in 30 minutes?

INGREDIENTS

2 chicken thighs or breasts

12 Oz chopped Butternut squash (about 2 ½ cups)

1 tablespoon + 2 teaspoons coconut oil

6 cups mixed greens

1 avocado, chopped

¼ cup tahini

1 tablespoon lemon juice

1 tablespoon apple cider vinegar

3 tablespoons water

Salt

Pepper

Garlic powder

INSTRUCTIONS

1.   Preheat oven to 425 degrees. Place butternut squash on a baking sheet. Toss with 2 teaspoons of melted coconut oil, ½ teaspoon salt, ¼ teaspoon pepper & ¼ teaspoon garlic powder. Roast in the oven for 25 minutes, tossing around halfway through.

2.   Take your chicken and sprinkle both sides with salt, pepper and garlic powder. Place a large saute pan over medium-high heat. Add 1 tablespoon of coconut oil and let heat up for about 30 seconds. Then add chicken and cook for 3-4 minutes on each side, depending on how thick they are (If they are thick I suggest pounding them down a bit so they all have an even thickness). Set chicken aside.

3.   In a small bowl, combine tahini, lemon juice, apple cider vinegar, water, ½ teaspoon salt, ¼ teaspoon pepper & ¼ teaspoon garlic powder. Toss a couple of tablespoons of dressing over the greens in a large bowl until evenly coated.

4.   To assemble bowl, add lettuce and top with butternut squash, chopped chicken, and avocado pieces. Drizzle more tahini dressing on top and enjoy.

MANGO CHICKEN WITH COCONUT CAULIFLOWER RICE

This recipe makes two clever swaps: The first is cauliflower "rice" instead of the usual white grain, and the second is tapioca flour as breading for the chicken. Add ginger and trusty coconut amino's to round out this healthier version of a takeout classic. Genius.

INGREDIENTS

For the sauce:

2 1/2 tsp Coconut oil dividend

1 1/2 tsp Fresh ginger minced

1 tsp Garlic, minced

1/2 tsp Habanero pepper, minced

3/4 Cup Orange Mango or Mango, Juice (100% pure juice)

1/2 Tbsp Coconut amino

1 tsp Tapioca flour

For the chicken:

3 Tbsp Tapioca flour

8 oz Chicken breast patted dry and cut into one-inch cubes

Salt + Pepper

2 Tbsp Coconut Oil

For the cauliflower rice:

3 Cups Cauliflower, cut into bite-sized pieces

2 tsp Coconut oil

2 Tbsp Unsweetened coconut flakes

For garnish:

1/2 a Large mango, cut into cubes

Roughly chopped cilantro

Diced Green Onion

Toasted sesame seeds

INSTRUCTIONS

1.   In a medium pot over medium heat, melt 1 1/2 tsp of the coconut oil for the sauce. Add the ginger, garlic and Habanero pepper and cook until fragrant, about 1 minute.

2.   Add in the juice and coconut amino's. Raise the temperature to high heat and bring to a boil. Additionally, place the tapioca flour in a small bowl.

3.   Once the liquid comes to a boil, add 2 tsp of it to the bowl with the tapioca flour and whisk until smooth. While stirring constantly, pour the tapioca mixture into the sauce and boil for 2 minutes.

4.   After the sauce as boiled, reduce the heat to medium-low and simmer, stirring frequently, until the sauce reduces by about 1/4 and becomes shiny about 6-7 minutes. Transfer to a large bowl to let it cool and thicken while you make the chicken.

5.   Place the tapioca flour into a large ziplock bag and season the cubed chicken with salt and pepper. Add the chicken in the bag and shake around until evenly coated with the flour.

6.   In a medium pan, heat 1 Tbsp of the coconut oil over medium-high heat. Place half of the chicken into the pan, being careful not to crowd it, and cook until golden brown, about 2-3 minutes. Flip and repeat. Transfer the chicken to a paper towel-lined plate and blot off an excess oil. Repeat

with the remaining chicken. If the chicken starts cooking too fast, turn the heat down a little bit.

7.   While the chicken cooks, place the cauliflower into a large food processor and process until broken down and "rice-like"

8.   Heat the 2 tsp of coconut oil up in a large pan over medium-high heat and add the cauliflower and coconut flakes. Cook until light golden brown, about 2-3 minutes. Cover, reduce the heat to medium and cook until the cauliflower is tender about 2-4 minutes.

9.   Transfer the chicken and mango cubes into the bowl with the sauce and toss until evenly coated.

10.   Divide the chicken and cauliflower between two plates and garnish with cilantro, green onion, and sesame seeds. This is also really good with just steamed cauliflower rice if you don't want to add the extra oil.

JALAPENO TURKEY BURGER

With gluten, dairy, and even ketchup out of the picture, you've got to get creative to make burgers taste good. Here, guacamole, a poached egg, and jalapeños up the ante.

INGREDIENTS

1 pound ground turkey (I prefer 85% lean, it has more fat, which makes for a better burger!) If your ground turkey has excess liquid, be sure to set on paper towels to remove the juices.

½-3/4 of one jalapeño pepper, minced

1 medium size shallot, peeled and minced

Zest and of one lime, and 2 teaspoon lime juice

2 Tablespoon chopped cilantro

1 teaspoon paprika

1 teaspoon cumin

½ a teaspoon sea salt

½ teaspoon black pepper

Guacamole

Pico de Gallo

Poached Egg (optional)

INSTRUCTIONS

1.   Note: The ground turkey to buy is the consistency of hamburger. If yours seems to have extra liquid, set on paper towels to drain juices.

2.   Place turkey, herbs, spices and lime in a bowl and use hands to mix well.

3.   Form into four patties.

4.   Place pan on medium heat.

5.   Add olive oil to the bottom of the pan.

6.   When the pan is hot, place patties in pan and cook for about 5 minutes each side or until cooked through.

7.   Top with guacamole, Pico de Gallo, and poached egg if desired.

GRILLED SALMON WITH MANGO SALSA

No restrictions on healthy fats while on the Whole Diet! And thank goodness for that, because we have a feeling you wouldn't be able to stay away from this cholesterol-slashing, omega-packed dish. Flaky salmon with a chunky mango salsa? Irresistible.

INGREDIENTS

4 6-ounce salmon fillets

1 teaspoon garlic powder

1 teaspoon chili powder

Salt and pepper to taste

Juice of 1 lime

Mango salsa

2-3 mangos, diced

½ red pepper,

½ red onion, diced

1 small jalapeño, seeded and finely chopped

¼ cup packed cilantro leaves, roughly chopped

INSTRUCTIONS

1.   In a medium bowl, stir together mangoes, red peppers, onions, jalapeños, and cilantro. Set aside until ready to use.

2.   Stir together garlic powder, chili powder, and salt and pepper (I used about a ½ teaspoon each). Rub mixture onto salmon fillets. Grill over medium heat for 6-8 minutes on each side.

3.   Squeeze fresh lime juice over grilled salmon, then top with mango salsa and serve.

WHITEFISH FILLET WITH BRAISED FENNEL

Not counting salt and pepper, there are only three ingredients in this dish. Plus the large fillet of white fish makes for a super-filling protein source. Pair it with fennel; the vitamin C-heavy cousin of carrots; for an easy but elegant dinner.

INGREDIENTS

White Fish Fillet

1 large white fish fillet per person

Pinch Himalayan or fine sea salt

Few grinds freshly cracked black pepper

The juice of half a lemon or lime

Braised Fennel

½ large fennel bulb per person

Pinch Himalayan or fine sea salt

Few grinds freshly cracked black pepper

INSTRUCTIONS

For the Braised Fennel

1.   Cut off the stalks from the fennel bulbs and cut each bulb lengthwise into 6 thick slices.

2.   It's important that you do not remove the core otherwise, the slices will fall apart.

3.   Season each fennel slice with a little bit of salt and pepper.

4.   In a large, heavy skillet, heat a little bit of olive oil or coconut oil over medium-high heat until your pan gets really hot. Add the fennel slices and cook until nice and brown, then flip the slices and cook the other side.

5.   Lower the heat, cover and continue cooking for about 6-8 minutes, until the fennel is good and tender.

For the fish fillets

1.   Pat the fish dry and season with a little bit of salt and pepper.

2.   Heat a little bit of olive or coconut oil in a medium non-stick skillet, over medium-high heat. When the pan is hot enough, add fillets and cook until it starts to form a little bit of a brown crust and flesh turns almost completely opaque. Very delicately flip the fillets and continue cooking until fish is cooked all the way through and no longer translucent. This should take about 1½ to 2 minutes per side, depending on thickness.

3.   Sprinkle with lemon or lime juice and transfer to dinner plates

4.   Serve with braised fennel, loaded coleslaw, and fresh greens.

SHRIMP AND ASPARAGUS STIR-FRY

Coconut oil lends an appropriately tropical taste (not to mention antimicrobial benefits) to the shrimp in this light, brothy stir-fry. Simply seasoned with lemon, ginger, and garlic, it's the 15-minute clean meal you can throw together with no matter how tired you are after a busy day.

INGREDIENTS

2tablespoonscoconut oil

1poundshrimp, peeled

1bundleasparagus, chopped

2tablespoonslemon juice

4clovesgarlic, minced

1/2teaspoonground ginger

2/3cupbroth

INSTRUCTIONS

1.   Heat the fat in a skillet over medium-high heat.

2.   Add the shrimp, asparagus, lemon juice, garlic, and ginger to the pan.

3.   Cook about 2 minutes, then stir and cook another 2 minutes.

4.   Add the broth and simmer until the asparagus is tender and the shrimp is pink 2-4 minutes.

BLACKENED CAJUN MAHI MAHI

This recipe calls for a few more spices than you might normally stock, but each will go a long way in flavoring the fish. And yes, you'll undoubtedly find yourself using them for other recipes while on the Whole Diet. Use them here for a rub to slather onto brain power-enhancing mahi-mahi fillets before the fish gets seared and topped with sliced avocado.

INGREDIENTS

Blacked Cajun Spice Rub

1 teaspoon dried parsley

1 teaspoon dried oregano

1 teaspoon dried thyme

1 teaspoon smoked paprika

½ teaspoon cayenne pepper*

½ teaspoon onion powder

½ teaspoon garlic powder

½ teaspoon salt

½ teaspoon pepper

Blackened Cajun Mahi Mahi

(2) 6oz wild caught Mahi filets, thawed and patted dry

1 tablespoon coconut oil

1 avocado, sliced

Lime wedges for serving

INSTRUCTIONS

1. Make the spice rub by combining all the dried spices on a plate and stirring with a fork to combine.

2. Heat a medium size skillet over medium-high heat. While it is heating up, dredge the fish fillets in the spice rub and coat evenly. When the pan is warm, add the coconut oil, and cook the spice-rubbed fish until cooked thru. Cooking time will depend on the thickness of your fish. Typically about 3 to 4 minutes per side.

3.   Serve warm. Top with sliced avocado and wedges of lime.

1/2 teaspoon cayenne pepper will make this mildly spicy. If you like it spicier, feel free to add more. If you are heat sensitive, add less or even leave it out so it is more kid friendly.

SKILLET BEEF FAJITAS

This homey Tex-Mex favorite is packed with veggies and a spicy kick. Throw everything in a skillet, and you'll be done in 30 minutes. Just make sure your broth of choice is Whole Diet approved (or if you're game, make it from scratch).

INGREDIENTS
Steak:
1½ lb flank steak, sliced into thin ribbons against the grain
1 lime, juiced
½ teaspoon chili powder
¼ teaspoon of ground cayenne red pepper
⅛ teaspoon cumin
⅛ teaspoon paprika
⅛ teaspoon ground black pepper

½ teaspoon dried oregano

½ teaspoon Sea salt

¼ teaspoon ground black pepper

Vegetables:

2 tablespoon organic coconut oil

1 yellow bell pepper, trimmed, deseeded and sliced

1 red bell pepper, trimmed, deseeded and sliced

1 yellow onion, trimmed, peeled and sliced into thin slices

1 garlic clove, minced

5 ounces shiitake mushrooms

2 green onions, green part, sliced

1 cup vegetable broth

1 jalapeno, seeded and sliced thinly {leave the seeds if you like it HOT}

¼ cup chopped cilantro

1 avocado, peeled, seeded and thinly sliced

INSTRUCTIONS

1.   Place steak, lime juice and spices in a large bowl and toss together until steak is evenly coated.

2.   Set aside.

3.   Place a large, heavy skillet over medium-high heat, I used cast-iron. Add coconut oil to the pan and when melted add steak.

4.   Try to lay steak out so that it is in a single layer on the pan.

5.   Let steak sear 3-4 minutes, flip and cook the other side of steak for an additional 3-4 minutes, you want the outside to be completely seared. Remove steak from pan and set aside on a plate.

6.   Add onions, peppers, garlic and mushrooms to pan, tossing to coat. There should be enough juice from the steak to toss and coat your veggies. If not, add about ¼ cup of your vegetable broth. Try to scrape any excess brown bits that are stuck to the bottom of the pan. Toss your veggies until they start to soften, about 5 minutes. Add green onion, jalapeño, vegetable broth, steak and any juices that collected on the plate.

7.   Toss and cook for an additional 5-8 minutes.

8.   Remove from heat, toss cilantro on top as well as sliced avocado and additional jalapeño slices if you like.

9.   Serve with rice, fajitas or lettuce cups

SWEET POTATO AND PINEAPPLE BEEF BOWLS

A hearty salad bowl can be the perfect quick fix when you don't feel like getting out the pots and pans. This one gets its sweetness from pineapple and mango. Just be sure you opt for the real thing (not the canned versions) to avoid added sugars.

INGREDIENTS

For the Sweet Potato

3-4 large sweet potatoes, cut into 1-inch pieces

2 tablespoons olive oil

½ teaspoon salt

For the Pineapple Beef

1 tablespoon olive oil

1 pound lean ground beef (grass-fed if possible)

1 can 8oz crushed pineapple

1 teaspoon cumin

1 teaspoon garlic powder

1 teaspoon mild chili powder

½ teaspoon salt

For the Salsa

1 large mango, diced

2 avocados, diced

1 lime, juiced

¼ cup cilantro

¼ teaspoon salt

For the Bowls

5 oz baby spinach

Hot sauce (optional)

INSTRUCTIONS

1.   Heat the oven to 400F.

2.   Toss the sweet potatoes, 2 tablespoons olive oil, and ½ teaspoon salt together on a sheet pan.

3.   Roast for 15 minutes, flip the potatoes, then roast an additional 15 minutes or until golden brown and tender.

4.   Heat 1 tablespoon olive oil in a large saute pan. Add the beef, stirring to break into chunks. Sprinkle with cumin,

garlic powder, mild chile powder, and ½ teaspoon salt. Cook 5-8 minutes or until the beef is browned and cooked through. Drain any extra fat, then add the pineapple and stir to combine. Turn the heat to low until ready to serve.

5.   Combine the mango, avocado, lime juice, cilantro, and salt in a large bowl. Stir to combine.

6.   Place the spinach, pineapple beef, and sweet potatoes in a bowl. Top with the mango, avocado salsa and hot sauce to taste.

HEARTY VEGETABLE SOUP

With only one tablespoon of olive oil in the entire six-serving recipe, this may be a lower fat dish, but it's no "diet" soup. Packed with potatoes, lean ground beef, and chunky tomato sauce, it's a filling and nutritious dinner that's also easy to make in big batches.

INGREDIENTS:

1 Tablespoon olive oil

1 teaspoon minced garlic

1 to 1 1/2 pound lean ground beef or turkey

1/2 cup chopped onion

2 small potatoes or sweet potatoes, peeled and diced (can also substitute with cauliflower)

1 cup chopped celery

1 cup chopped carrots

1 (14.5 ounces) can rotel

1 (15 ounces) can tomato sauce

1 cup water

1 Tablespoon balsamic vinegar

1 - 2 teaspoons chili powder, more or less to taste

1/2 teaspoon kosher salt

1/2 teaspoon ground black pepper

3 tomatoes, diced (or substitute with 1-14 ounce can)

INSTRUCTIONS

1.   Heat the oil in a large pot over medium heat. Add the chopped onions and cook for 2 minutes. Stir in the garlic and cook for an additional 1 minute. Next, stir in the ground beef and cook until browned. Drain any remaining fat.

2.   Stir in potatoes, celery, and carrots, rotel, tomato sauce and water. Bring to a light simmer and then stir in the balsamic vinegar, chili powder, salt, pepper, and tomatoes.

3.   Reduce the heat to low and let simmer for about 30-45 minutes (or until the potatoes and carrots are forks tender), stirring occasionally.

4.   Top with fresh basil if desired.

PORK ROAST WITH SWEET POTATOES, APPLES, AND ONION

Instead of sugary or preservative-laden applesauce, this Whole Diet makeover of the favorite pork and apple combo uses fresh chunks of the fruit, roasting it for a naturally sweet side to the protein. With diced sweet potato pitching in for some additional carb action, this meaty dish scores plenty of produce points.

INGREDIENTS

2 1/2 pound pork roast

2-4 apples, quartered (used small gala, so used 4 apples, but if you use a larger apple like pink, lady or granny smith, I would only use 2)

2 sweet potatoes, cut into wedges

1 sweet onion, sliced

1/2 teaspoon sweet paprika

1/4 teaspoon cumin

1/4 teaspoon chili powder

Salt and pepper to taste

Olive oil (about 1/4 cup) enough to coat

INSTRUCTIONS

1.   Preheat broiler to 500.

2.   Rub pork with olive oil and season with salt and pepper.

3.   Place on sheet tray and broil for 15 minutes, flipping halfway through cooking time (to get a nice color of meat).

4.   Meanwhile, chop apples, sweet potatoes, and onions. Toss in oil and spices.

5.   Arrange on sheet tray around the pork roast.

6.   Turn oven to down 450, and roast for 20-30 minutes, until apples and sweet potatoes are tender and meat reaches 120 degrees. This is a preference, most might say to cook for 140, but that is how you get dry pork. Allow the meat to rest at least 10 minutes before slicing and it will continue to cook and will be juicy! Return sliced pork and juices to the pan.

7.   Serve sliced pork with sweet potatoes, apples, onions and a simple salad.

BALSAMIC AND BASIL MARINATED STEAK WITH ROASTED RED PEPPER PESTO

With just 10 main ingredients, skirt steak gets elevated from mere hunks of meat to seared strips loaded with flavor—and a ton of muscle-aiding iron. Soaked in a tangy marinade before generous dollops of the zippy (and nondairy!) red pepper pesto spoon on top.

INGREDIENTS

Steak Marinade

Balsamic basil marinated steak

1lb skirt steak (any steak)

1/4 cup balsamic vinegar

2 tbsp avocados or olive oil

1/4 cup fresh chopped basil (or 1 tbsp dried basil) 1 tbsp fresh minced garlic (or 1 tsp garlic powder

1 tsp pepper

1 tsp salt

1 tsp onion powder

Roasted Red Pepper Pesto

1/2 cup fresh basil, packed

1/2 cup roasted red peppers

1/4 cup pine nuts

1/4 cup olive oil

1 large garlic clove

1/2 tsp salt

1/2 tsp pepper

INSTRUCTIONS

1.   Marinate steak in a gallon sized plastic bag or Tupperware overnight or a minimum of 4 hours.

2.   Pan sear a steak in ghee or grill until cooked to your preference.

3.   While steak is cooking, prepare pesto.

4.   Add all pesto ingredients to food processor and pulse until combined into a pesto texture.

5.   Serve pesto on top of cooked steak.

LAMB, MINT CHIMICHURRI, AND BUTTERNUT RICE

Cauliflower isn't the only veggie you can morph into rice-like granules! Butternut squash also makes an awesome substitute for the grain. Here it's made all buttery and wonderful with the addition of ghee (yup, enjoy ghee with glee!) and then topped with grilled lamb and drizzled with a fresh, herby chimichurri. This is dinner party-worthy stuff.

INGREDIENTS

2 pounds boneless lamb loin

Kosher salt

Freshly ground pepper

1 tbsp. olive oil

1 cup firmly packed fresh mint leaves

½ cup firmly packed flat-leaf parsley

2 garlic cloves, chopped

1 tsp. dried crushed red pepper

½ cup olive oil

⅓ cup red wine vinegar

1 butternut squash, peeled, seeded and roughly chopped (approximately 4 cups)

1 tablespoon ghee

3 cups beef broth

INSTRUCTIONS

1.   Make the chimichurri: put parsley, mint, garlic, red pepper flakes, olive oil and red wine vinegar in the bowl of a food processor and pulse 15-20 times until blended but not pureed. Pour into a bowl, cover and set aside.

2.   Prep the squash: Clean out the bowl of the food processor and add squash. Pulse 5-10 times until the squash resembles the size of rice. Set aside.

3.   Light charcoal grill or preheat a gas grill to 350-400 degrees. Add lamb loins and cover the grill. Grill for approximately 5 minutes on one side, then flip over and grill the other side approximately 3-5 minutes until the internal temp of the lamb reaches 130 degrees for medium rare.

4.   Remove loins from the grill, cover loosely with foil and let rest 5-7 minutes.

5.   While the lamb is resting, pour squash into a medium saucepan and add enough broth so the squash is just covered. Bring the squash mixture to a boil and add ghee. Reduce heat and simmer approximately 5-7 minutes until the

squash is tender. Drain squash in a colander or strainer and place in a serving dish.

6.   Cut lamb against the grain into ¼" thick slices, then drizzle chimichurri on top. Serve immediately.

TOMATO BASIL BEEF GOULASH WITH EGGPLANT

Trading in the dish's trademark paprika and caraway seeds for basil and garlic, and potatoes for eggplant. Whisking in the cream from the top of a can of coconut milk makes it extra luscious while keeping with the Whole Diet's no-dairy rule.

INGREDIENTS

2 tablespoons olive oil, divided

2 shallots, diced

4 garlic cloves, diced

1 lb ground beef

1 medium eggplant, cut into 1" cubes

1 (14oz) can diced tomatoes

⅓ cup fresh basil, diced

2 teaspoons salt

2 tablespoons tomato paste

¾ cup coconut cream (thick cream at the top of canned coconut milk)

INSTRUCTIONS

1.   Heat 1 tablespoon olive oil in a large saucepan over medium heat

2.   Add the shallots and garlic. Sauté for a few minute, until fragrant

3.   Add the ground beef and cook until brown

4.   In a separate saucepan, heat the other tablespoon of olive oil over medium heat and add the diced eggplant. Cook until soft, around 5 minutes

5.   Once the beef is browned, drain any excess grease, add the diced tomatoes (with juice), basil, and salt. Stir to combine, then add the coconut cream, tomato paste, and eggplant

6.   Serve immediately and garnish with more fresh basil

PALEO EGGS IN HELL

Eating clean, real foods on the Whole Diet doesn't mean splurging on pricey or obscure ingredients. Take this dinner, which turns a modest ingredient list into a protein-rich dish that, contrary to its name, tastes pretty heavenly.

INGREDIENTS

1 (28 oz) can diced tomatoes

1 tablespoon olive oil

1/2 white onion, diced

2 teaspoons red pepper flakes

1 tablespoon Italian seasoning

1/2 teaspoon salt

4 eggs

Parsley, for serving (optional)

INSTRUCTIONS

1.   In a large cast iron skillet or Dutch oven, heat 1 tablespoon of olive oil over medium-high heat. Sauté the onion until soft, about 4 minutes. Stir in the red pepper flakes, salt, and Italian seasoning and stir until fragrant, about 1 minute.

2.   Pour in the tomatoes and bring to a simmer for about 5 minutes. Make 4 divots in the sauce and crack an egg in each. Reduce the heat to low and cover. Cook for 3-5 minutes until the egg whites are set, but the yolk is still runny. Sprinkle with parsley and serve.

ZUCCHINI NOODLES WITH EVERYTHING PESTO AND FRIED EGGS

If spiralized zucchini never seemed like an adequate pasta alternative before, maybe this recipe will convince you. Lathered in a dairy-free pesto and topped with a fried egg, the noodles are every bit as tasty as real spaghetti, but with none of the gluten and a fraction of the carbs.

INGREDIENTS

For the everything pesto

1/4 Cup + 2 Tbsp Pine nuts toasted

1 Cup Lightly packed fresh herbs of choice, used basil

2 Scallions, trimmed and roughly chopped

1 clove Garlic, crushed

1/4 tsp Flaky sea salt or more to taste

3 Tbsp Extra-virgin olive oil

1 tsp Fresh lime or lemon juice

For the squash noodles and fried eggs

2 pounds of 3 zucchini, summer squash or cousa squash, julienned or spiralized (I used zucchini)

1/2 tsp Flaky sea salt or more to taste

3 tsp Ghee or extra-virgin olive oil

Freshly ground black pepper

2 Large eggs

INSTRUCTIONS

To make the everything pesto:

1.   Pulse 1/4 cup of the pine nuts, the herbs, scallion, garlic and salt in a food processor until coarsely chopped. Add the olive oil and lime juice and pulse again, scraping down the sides of the bowl as needed. Taste the pesto and add more salt if desired.

To make the squash noodles and fried eggs:

1.   Put the squash in a colander lined with paper towels. Toss with 1/2 tsp of salt and set aside for a few minutes, so the salt can draw some of the moisture out of the squash

2.   Heat 1 tsp of the ghee in a large skillet with a lid over medium-high heat. Add the squash noodles and cook, tossing frequently, until cooked to your liking. Take it off the heat and add the pesto. Toss to combine, and season with salt and pepper to taste. Cover the skillet to keep the noodles, hot while you make the eggs.

3.   Heat the remaining 2 tsp of ghee in a medium-sized skillet over medium heat, and fry the eggs until cooked to your liking.

4.   Divide the noodles between 2 plates. Top each pile of noodles with a fried egg and 1 Tablespoon of pine nuts. Serve immediately.

SLOW COOKER RATATOUILLE SOUP

With a whopping eight different veggies, this may as well be called "the one-stop stew for your daily recommended fiber and vitamin intake" (although "ratatouille soup" sounds much more appetizing). The produce is cooked down in a mix of its own juices and fruity olive oil, yielding a large batch that will have dinner covered for days.

INGREDIENTS

8 tomatoes, boiled, skinned and chopped

2 red bell peppers (chopped)

2 yellow bell peppers (chopped)

2 green bell peppers (chopped)

2 small zucchini (chopped)

1 yellow squash (chopped)

1 eggplant (peeled and cubed)

1 yellow onion (chopped)

1/4 cup olive oil

2 tsp minced garlic

2 T fresh basil, chopped

2 T fresh parsley

Sea salt to taste

INSTRUCTIONS

Throw everything in a slow cooker and cook for at least 6 hours. Cook on high for the first hour and then turn down to low for the remaining hours. Feel free to cook it longer than 6 hours if you like. I think the longer a soup cook, the more the flavors develop.

Notes: To peel the tomatoes, core them and place them in a saucepan of boiling water. After a minute or two, pull them out and place them in an ice water bath. The skin should easily come off. You can try leaving the skins on for this soup, but they may get tough while cooking so long. Don't throw the skins away, though. You can save them with all your other scraps for homemade vegetable broth. Enjoy!

SWEET POTATO AND KALE GRATIN

This gratin may be grain-free, gluten-free, and dairy-free, but it makes no compromises when it comes to flavor. A coconut milk-based cream sauce, fragrant with nutmeg, and an entire head of garlic. Gets slathered generously between layers of sweet potato disks and kale for a one-pan dinner that's light and decadent all at once.

INSTRUCTIONS

For the roasted garlic

1 head garlic

1/2 teaspoon olive oil

For the gratin:

4 tablespoons ghee (melted) or olive oil, divided

1 bunch kale, tough stems removed, chopped

3 pounds sweet potatoes, peeled and thinly sliced into 1/8"
thick rounds

1/4 cup chicken or vegetable stock

1 and 1/2 cups coconut milk (one 14.5 ounce can)

1 teaspoon salt, or to taste

Freshly ground black pepper, to taste

1/4 teaspoon freshly grated nutmeg

INSTRUCTIONS

1.   Preheat the oven to 400. Cut the top off the head of
garlic so the tops of all the cloves are exposed, and drizzle
the cut side with the olive oil. Wrap the head in tinfoil and
place it right on your oven rack. Roast for about 45 minutes,
or until the cloves are very soft when squeezed or pierced
with a fork. Let cool for a few minutes, then squeeze each
clove out of its peel and set aside in a medium bowl.

2.   Meanwhile, steam the kale until wilted, 2-3 minutes.
You can use a metal strainer set over a saucepan of similar
size if you don't have a steamer. Put an inch or two of water
in the saucepan, bring it to a boil, set the strainer with the
kale on top, and cover. When the kale is wilted, set it aside
to cool.

3. Leave the oven at 400, and grease the bottom and sides of a 9×13" glass baking dish with two tablespoons of the ghee or olive oil.

4. Layer half the sweet potato slices in the bottom of the baking dish in overlapping rows. Squeeze the excess water from the kale and sprinkle it evenly on top of the sweet potatoes. Top with a little salt & pepper. Layer the remaining sweet potato slices on top of the kale.

5. Add the coconut milk, stock, salt, pepper, and nutmeg to the bowl with the roasted garlic. Process with an immersion blender (or transfer to your regular blender to puree) until smooth. Pour the sauce evenly over the potatoes, and drizzle the remaining two tablespoons of ghee or oil on top.

6. Cover the dish with tinfoil and bake for 25 minutes, then remove the tinfoil and bake for another 20-25 minutes, or until the sweet potatoes are tender. If you'd like to brown the top of your gratin a little more, set the oven to broil and place the gratin under the broiler for 1-2 minutes (don't walk away!). Let the gratin sit for 10 minutes before slicing and serving.

www.ingramcontent.com/pod-product-compliance
Lightning Source LLC
Chambersburg PA
CBHW070340220526
45467CB00001B/198